ANIMAL + CAT ANATOMY COLORING BOOK

SCAN THE CODE TO ACCESS YOUR FREE DIGITAL COPY

THIS BOOK BELONGS TO

_____

TABLE OF CONTENTS

TABLE OF CONTENTS

SECTION 1: ANIMAL CELL

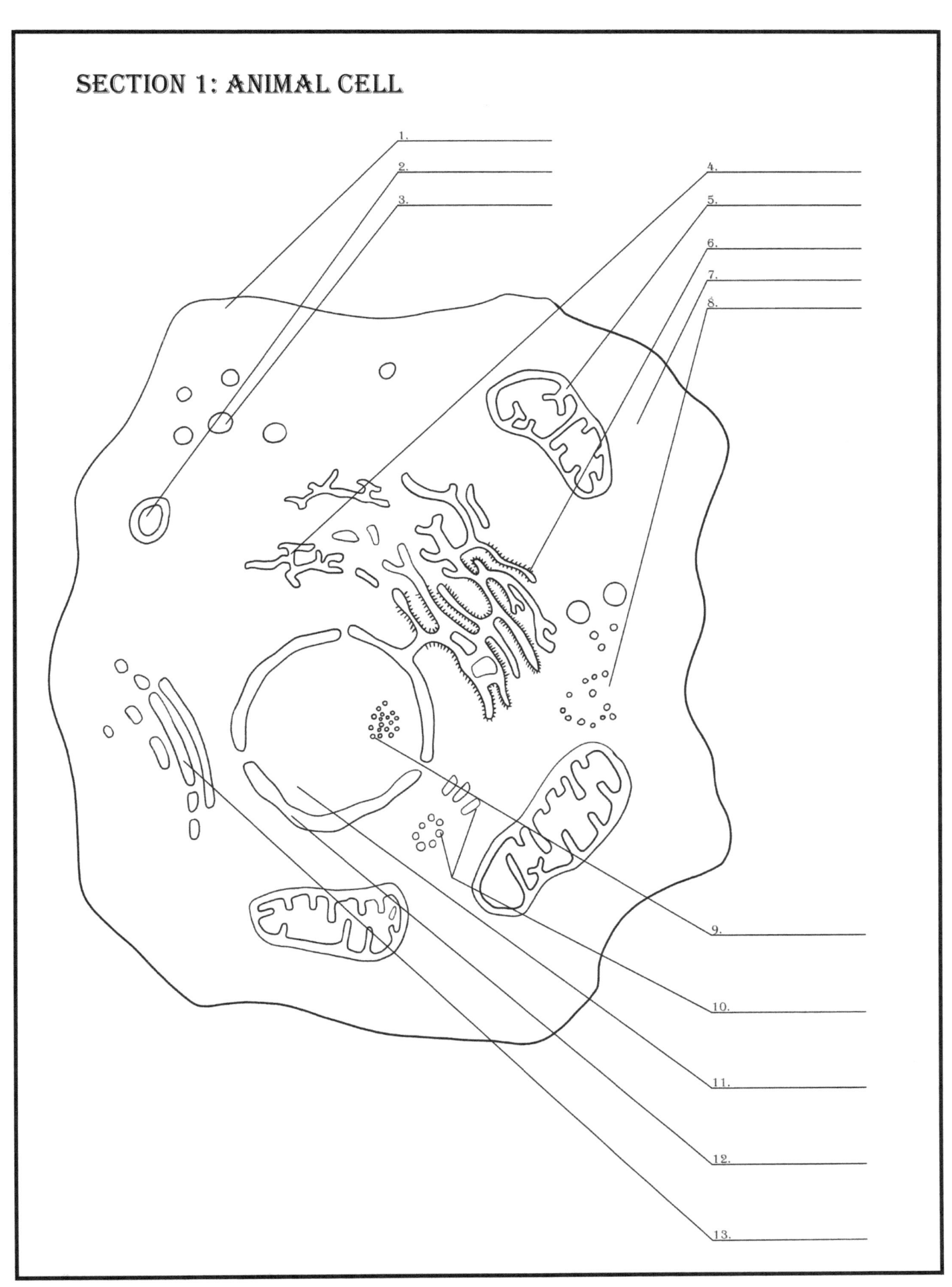

1. _____
2. _____
3. _____
4. _____
5. _____
6. _____
7. _____
8. _____
9. _____
10. _____
11. _____
12. _____
13. _____

SECTION 1: ANIMAL CELL

1. CELL MEMBRANE
2. LYSOSOME
3. VACUOLE
4. SMOOTH ENDOPLASMIC RETICULUM
5. MITOCHONDRION
6. ROUGH ENDOPLASMIC RETICULUM
7. CYTOPLASM
8. RIBOSOME
9. NUCLEOLUS
10. CETNRIOLES
11. CHROMATIN
12. NUCLEAR MEMBRANE
13. GOLGI APPARATUS

SECTION 2: FISH EXTERNAL FORM AND INTERNAL STRUCTURE

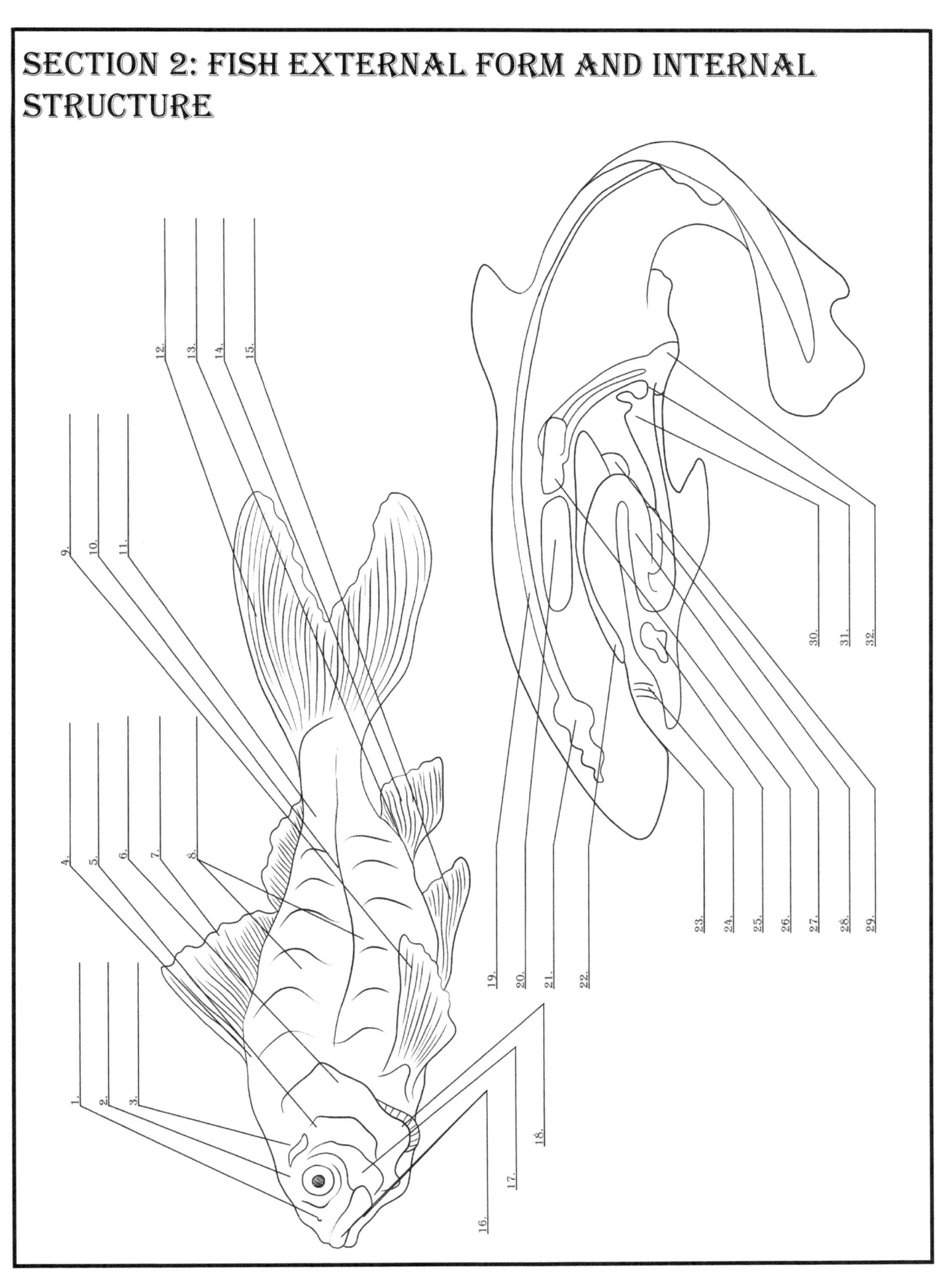

SECTION 2: FISH EXTERNAL FORM AND INTERNAL STRUCTURE

1. NOSTRIL
2. EYE
3. LEVATOR OCULI MUSCLE
4. DORSALIS MUSCLE
5. PREOPERCULUM
6. OPERCULUM (GIL COVER)
7. DORSAL FIN (ANTERIOR)
8. MYOTOME MUSCLES
9. PECTORAL FIN
10. LATERAL LINE
11. HORIZONTAL SEPTUM
12. CAUDAL FIN
13. ANUS
14. ANAL FIN
15. PELVIC FIN
16. MAXILLA
17. ABDUCTOR MANDIBULAE
18. BRACHIOSTEGALS
19. SPINAL CORD
20. OVARY
21. BRAIN
22. LIVER
23. MOUTH
24. GILL SLIT
25. HEART
26. KIDNEY
27. STOMACH
28. PANCREAS
29. SPLEEN
30. INTESTINE
31. RECTUM
32. CLOACA

SECTION 3: FISH SKELETON

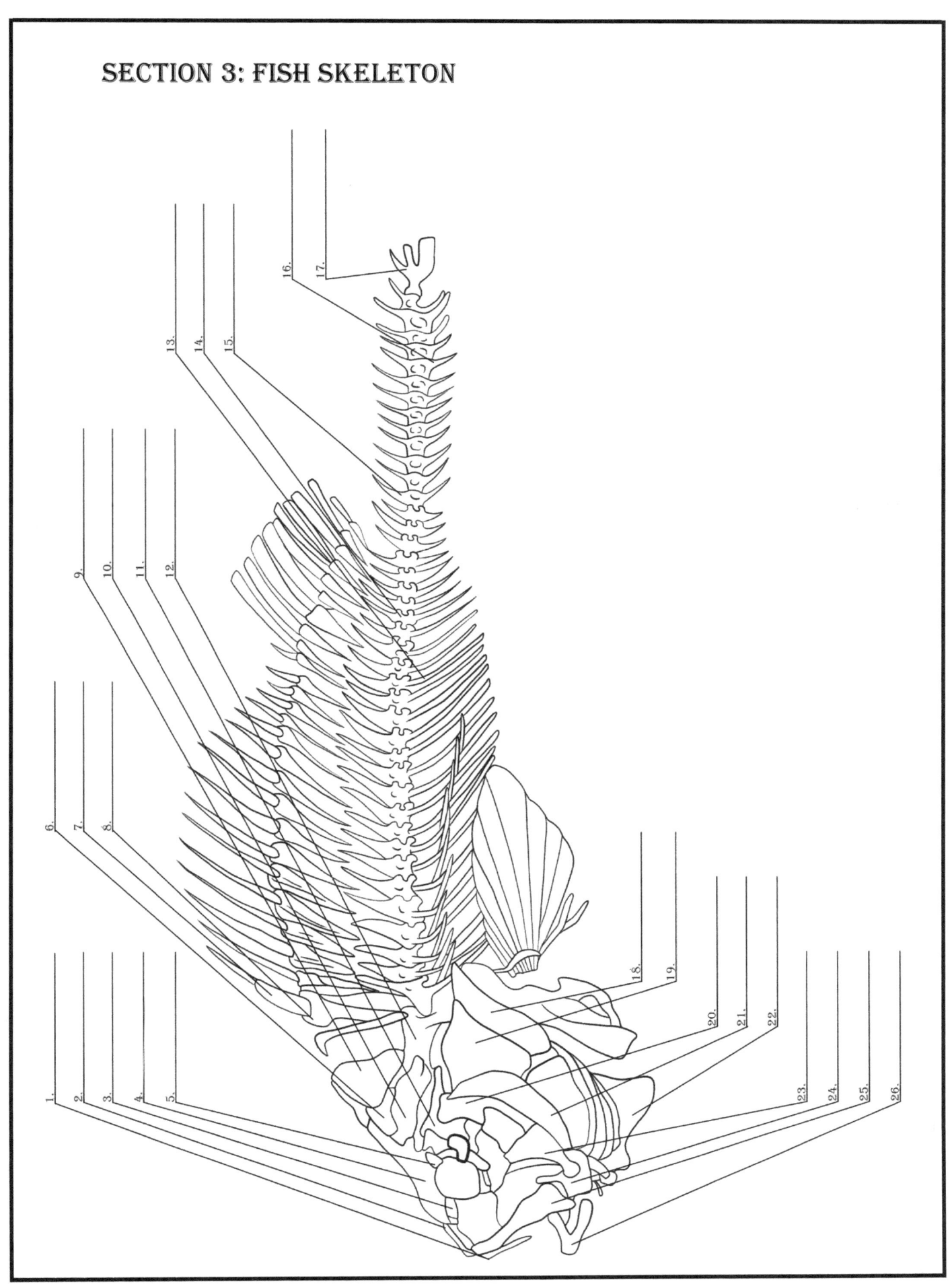

SECTION 3: FISH SKELETON

1. PREMAXILLA
2. ETHMOID
3. PREFRONTAL BONE
4. FRONTAL BONE
5. POSTFRONTAL BONE
6. PARIETAL BONE
7. DERMAL FIN RAY
8. BASAL AND RADIAL CARTILAGES
9. SUPRAOCCIPITAL BONE
10. EPIOTIC BONE
11. SQUAMOSAL BONE
12. PRETOTIC BONE
13. RIB
14. VERTEBRA
15. NEUTRAL SPINE
16. HEMAL SPINE
17. NOTOCHORD
18. SUBOPERCULAR BONE
19. OPERCULAR BONE
20. HYOMANDIBULAR BONE
21. PREOPERCULAR BONE
22. UROHYAL
23. QUADRATE BONE
24. ARTICULAR BONE
25. MAXILLA
26. DENARY BONE

SECTION 4: FROG EXTERNAL AND INTERNAL FORM

1. _____
2. _____
3. _____
4. _____
5. _____
6. _____
7. _____
8. _____
9. _____
10. _____
11. _____
12. _____
13. _____
14. _____
15. _____
16. _____

17. _____
18. _____
19. _____
20. _____
21. _____
22. _____
23. _____
24. _____
25. _____
26. _____

SECTION 4: FROG EXTERNAL AND INTERNAL FORM

1. ESOPHAGUS
2. CAROTID ARTERY
3. AORTIC ARCH
4. SUBCLAVIAN ARTERY
5. HEART
6. LUNGS
7. LIVER
8. STOMACH
9. FAT BODIES
10. KIDNEY
11. PANCREAS
12. SPLEEN
13. BLADDER
14. FEMORAL ARTERY
15. COMMON ILIAC ARTERY
16. SCIATIC ARTERY
17. EYE
18. EXTERNAL NOSTRIL
19. EAR DRUM
20. UPPER ARM
21. FINGER
22. WRIST
23. THIGH
24. SHANK
25. WEBBED TOE
26. ANKLE

SECTION 5: FROG SKELETON AND MUSCLES

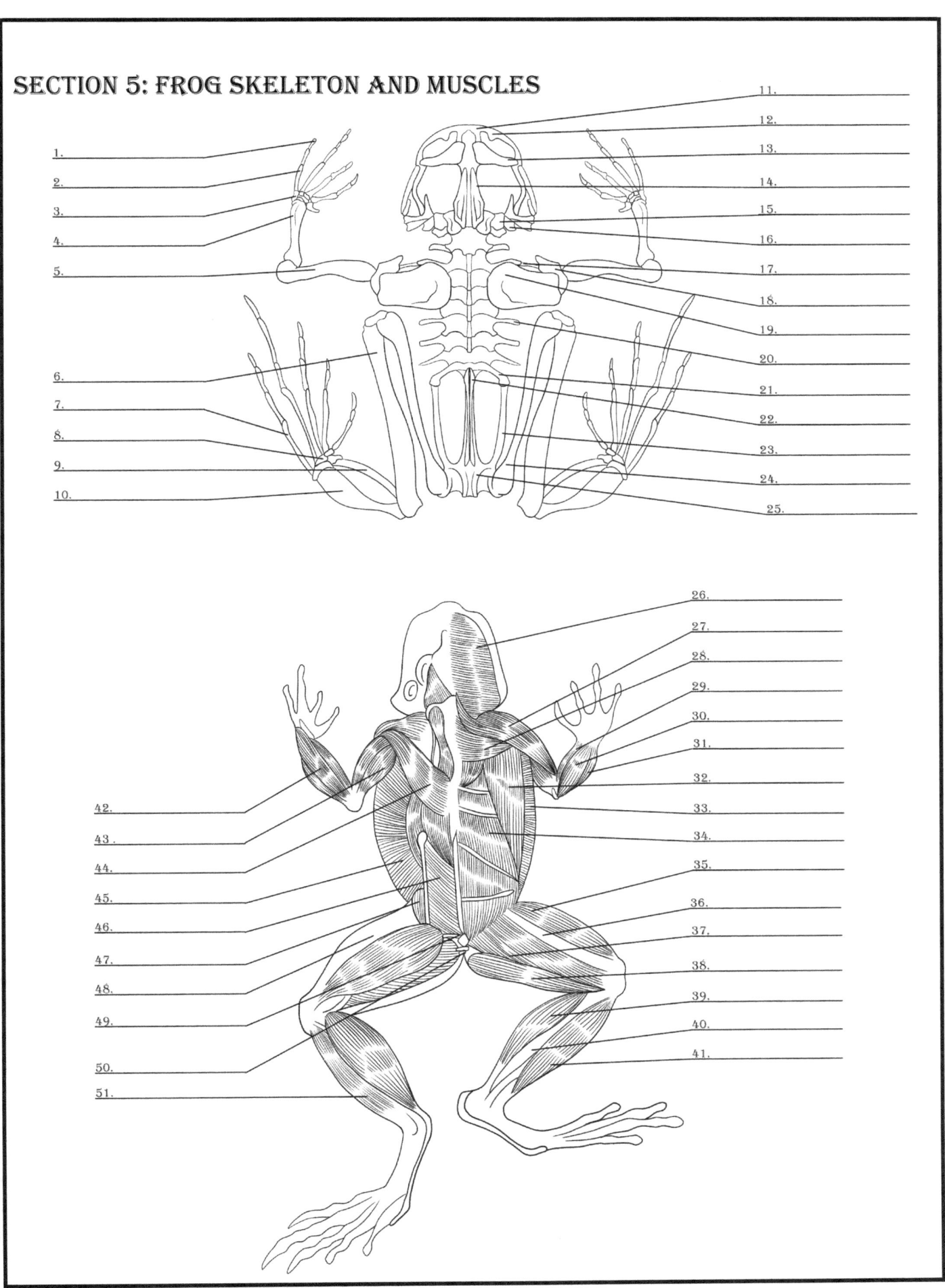

1. _____
2. _____
3. _____
4. _____
5. _____

6. _____
7. _____
8. _____
9. _____
10. _____

11. _____
12. _____
13. _____
14. _____
15. _____
16. _____
17. _____
18. _____
19. _____
20. _____
21. _____
22. _____
23. _____
24. _____
25. _____

26. _____
27. _____
28. _____
29. _____
30. _____
31. _____
32. _____
33. _____
34. _____
35. _____
36. _____
37. _____
38. _____
39. _____
40. _____
41. _____

42. _____
43. _____
44. _____
45. _____
46. _____
47. _____
48. _____
49. _____
50. _____
51. _____

SECTION 5: FROG SKELETON AND MUSCLES

1. PHALANGE
2. METACARPAL
3. CARPAL
4. RADIOULNA
5. HUMERUS
6. TIBIOFIBULA
7. METATARSAL
8. TARSAL
9. ASTRALAGUS
10. CALCANEUM
11. PREMAXILLA
12. MAXILLA
13. NASAL BONE
14. FRONTOPARIETAL BONE
15. PROOTIC BONE
16. EXOCCIPITAL BONE
17. CLAVICLE
18. CORACOID
19. SUPRASCAPULA
20. VERTEBRA
21. SACRAL VERTEBRA
22. UROSTYLE
23. ILIUM
24. FEMUR
25. ISCHIUM
26. MYLOHYOID
27. CORACORDIALIS
28. DELTOID
29. FLEXOR CARPI RADIALIS
30. FLEXOR PALMARIS
31. FLEXOR CARPI ULNARIS
32. PECTORALIS
33. OBLIQUUS EXTERNUS
34. RECTUS ABDOMINIS
35. TRICEPS FEMORIS
36. ABDUCTOR LONGUS
37. ABDUCTOR MAGNUS
38. GRACILIS MINOR
39. GASTROCNEMICUS
40. TIBIALIS POSTICUS
41. TIBIALIS ANTICUS LONGUS
42. DORSALISSCAPULAE
43. TRICEPS BRACHII
44. LATISSIMUS DORSI
45. OBLIQUUS INTERNUS
46. COCCYGEOILIACUS
47. ILIACUS EXTERNUS
48. ILIACUS
49. PYRIFORMIS
50. ANUS
51. PERONEUS

SECTION 6: LIZARD SKELETON AND INTERNAL STRUCTURE

1. _____
2. _____
3. _____
4. _____
5. _____

6. _____
7. _____
8. _____

9. _____
10. _____
11. _____
12. _____
13. _____
14. _____
15. _____
16. _____
17. _____

18. _____
19. _____
20. _____
21. _____

22. _____
23. _____
24. _____
25. _____
26. _____
27. _____

28. _____
29. _____
30. _____
31. _____
32. _____
33. _____
34. _____

35. _____
36. _____
37. _____
38. _____
39. _____
40. _____
41. _____

SECTION 6: LIZARD SKELETON AND INTERNAL STRUCTURE

1. SKULL
2. MANDIBLE
3. ATLAS
4. AXIS
5. CERVICAL VERTEBRAE
6. COSTAL CARTILAGE
7. PELVIS
8. SACRUM
9. SCAPULA
10. RIB
11. HUMERUS
12. STERNUM
13. RADIUS
14. ULNA
15. METACARPAL
16. PHALANGE
17. CLAW
18. FEMUR
19. PATELLA
20. TIBIA
21. FIBULA
22. CEREBRUM
23. OPTIC LOBE
24. CEREBELLUM
25. NOSTRIL
26. SPINAL CORD
27. TONGUE
28. TRACHEA
29. ESOPHAGUS
30. LIVER
31. LUNG
32. STOMACH
33. PANCREAS
34. DUODENUM
35. FUNNEL
36. OVARY
37. RECTUM
38. OVIDUCT
39. BLADDER
40. CLOACA
41. KIDNEY

SECTION 7: LIZARD MUSCLES

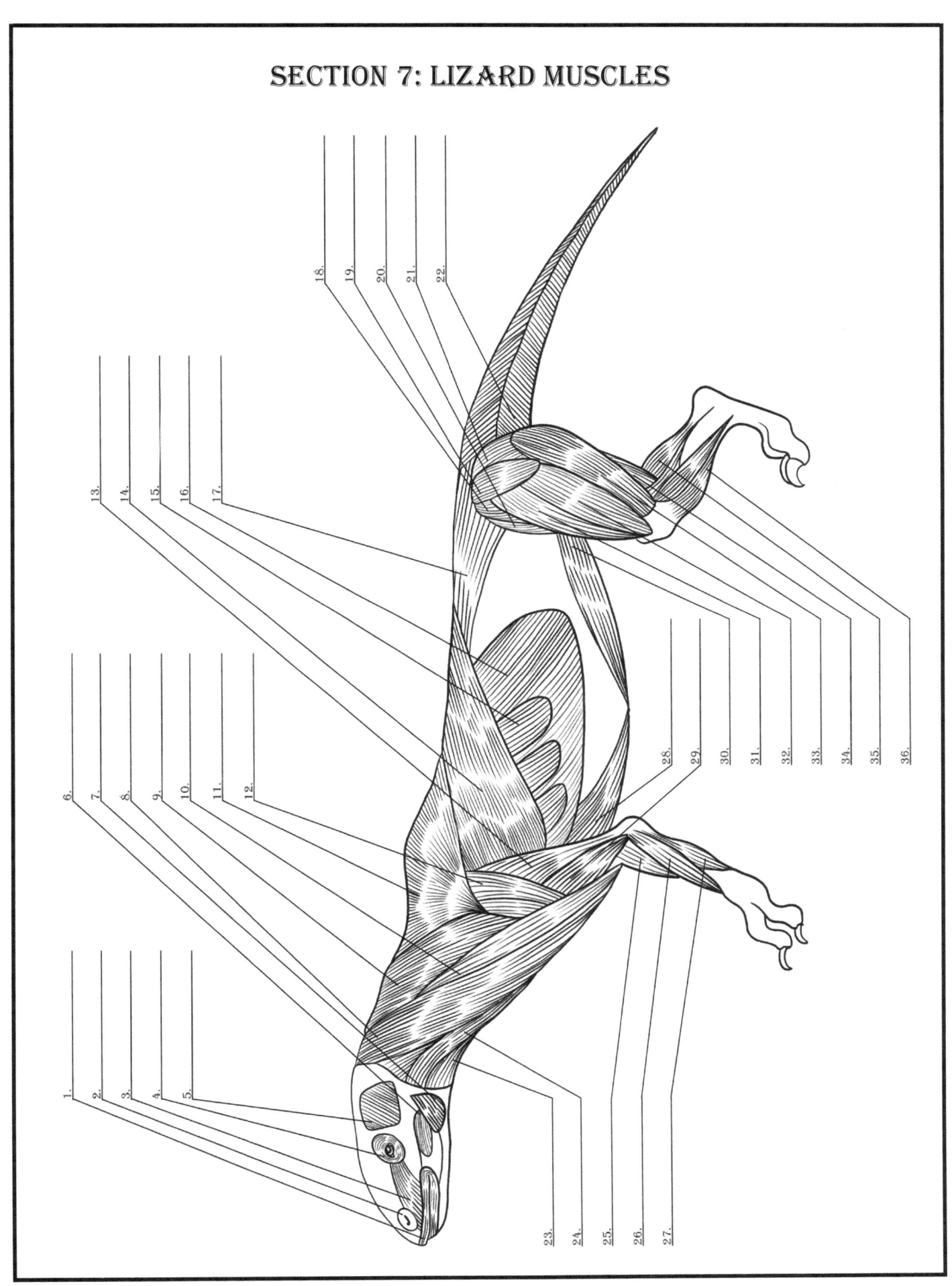

SECTION 7: LIZARD MUSCLES

1. ORBICULARIS ORIS
2. NOSTRIL
3. LEVATOR NASOLABIALIS
4. ORBICULARIS OCCULI
5. TEMPORALIS
6. ZYGOMATICUS
7. MASSETER
8. BRACHIOCEPUHALICUS
9. SPLENIUS
10. OMOTRANSVERSARIUS
11. TRAPEZIUS
12. DELTOID
13. TRICEPS
14. LATISSIMUS DORSI
15. SERRATUS VENTRALIS THORACIS
16. EXTERNAL ABDOMINAL OBLIQUE
17. LONGISSIMUS DORSI
18. RECTUS FEMORIS
19. GLUTEUS MEDIUS
20. SARTORIUS
21. GLUTEUS SUPERFICIAL
22. COCCYGEUS
23. STERNOTHYROHYOID
24. STERNOMANDIBULARIW
25. BRACHIORADIALIS
26. EXTENSOR DIGITORUM COMMUNIS
27. ULNARIS LATERALIS
28. PECTORALIS ASCENDENS
29. BRACHIALIS
30. RECTUS ABDOMINALIS
31. TENSOR FASCIALATAE
32. VASTUS LATRANS
33. BICEPS FEMORIS
34. SEMITENDINOSUS
35. GASTROCNEMICUS
36. EXTENSOR LATERALIS

SECTION 8: BIRD SKELETON

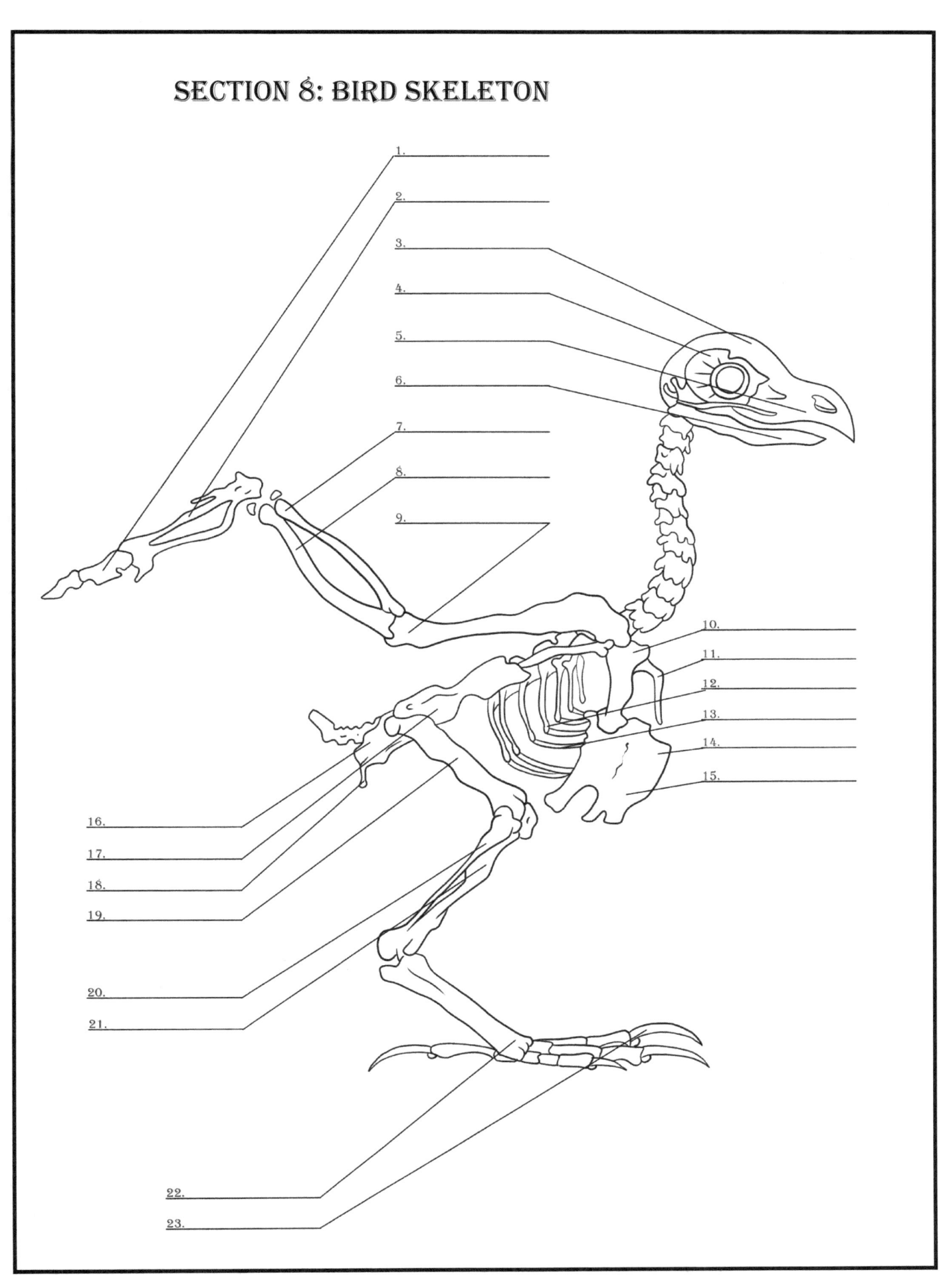

SECTION 8: BIRD SKELETON

1. PHALANGE
2. METACARPAL
3. CRANIUM
4. SCLERAL BONE (EYE SOCKET)
5. UPPER MANDIBLE
6. LOWER MANDIBLE
7. RADIUS
8. ULNA
9. HUMERUS
10. CORACOID
11. WURCULA (WISH BONE0
12. RIB
13. STERNAL RIB
14. KEEL
15. STERNUM
16. ISCHIUM
17. ILIUM
18. PUBIS
19. FEMUR
20. FIBULA
21. TIBIA
22. TARSOMETATARSUS
23. DIGIT

SECTION 9: BIRD INTERNAL STRUCTURE

1.
2.
3.
4.
5.
6.
7.
8.
9.
10.
11.
12.
13.
14.

15.
16.
17.
18.
19.
20.
21.
22.
23.
24.
25.
26.
27.
28.
29.
30.
31.
32.
33.
34.

SECTION 9: BIRD INTERNAL STRUCTURE

1. CEREBRUM
2. CEREBELLUM
3. SPINAL CORD
4. ESOPHAGUS
5. TRACHEA
6. KIDNEY
7. AIR SAC
8. STOMACH
9. GLIZZARD
10. INTESTINE
11. CLOACA
12. CROP
13. LUNG
14. LIVER
15. COMB
16. BRAIN
17. BEAK
18. ESOPHAGUS
19. TRACHEA
20. SPINAŁ CORD
21. OVARY
22. KIDNEY
23. OVIDUCT
24. CLOACA
25. LUNG
26. CROP
27. HEART
28. PROVENTRICULUS
29. GALL BLADDER
30. SPLEEN
31. GLIZZARD
32. MESENTERY
33. DUODENAL LOOP
34. PANCREAS

SECTION 10: BIRD EXTERNAL STRUCTURE

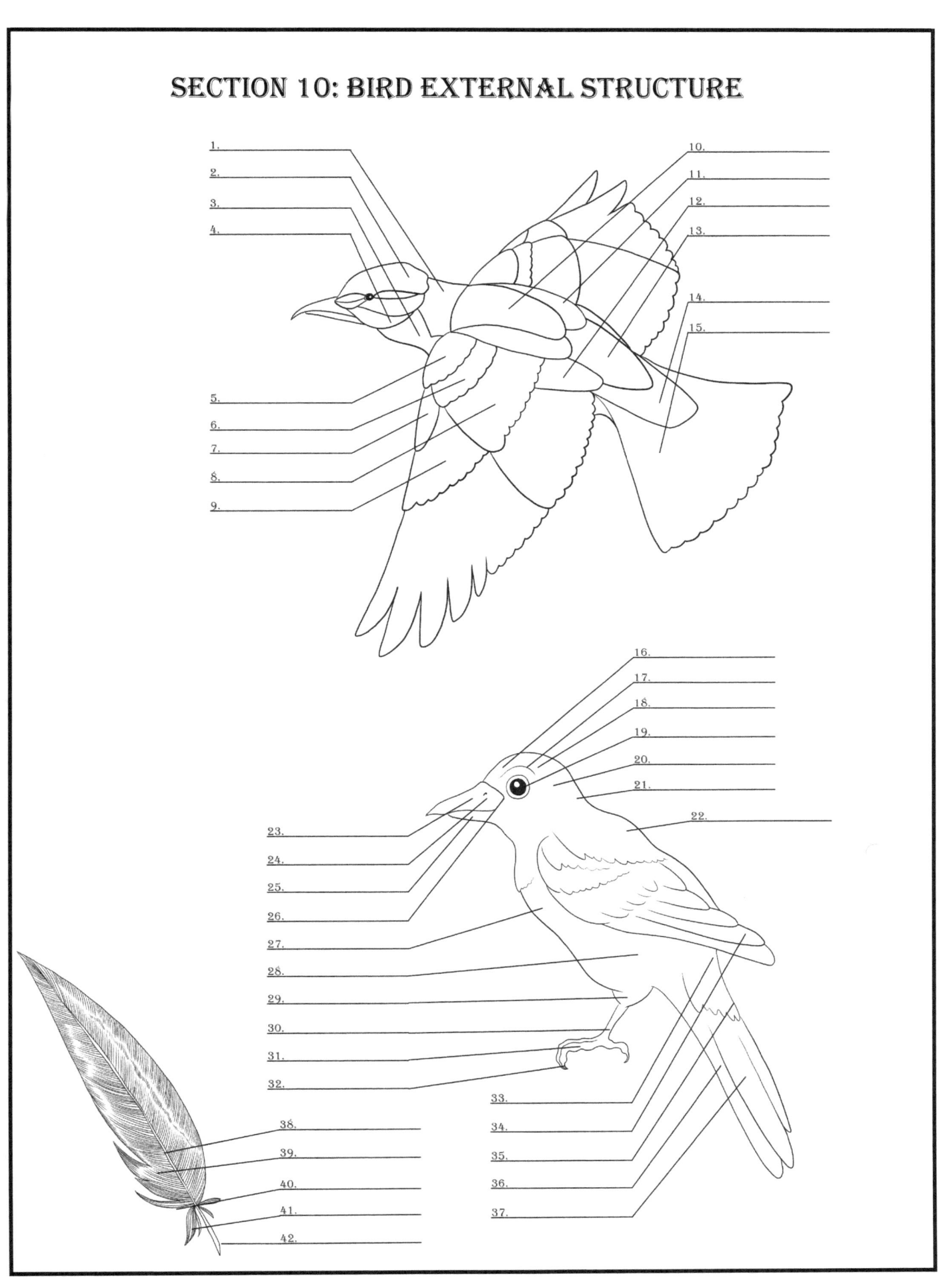

1.
2.
3.
4.
5.
6.
7.
8.
9.
10.
11.
12.
13.
14.
15.
16.
17.
18.
19.
20.
21.
22.
23.
24.
25.
26.
27.
28.
29.
30.
31.
32.
33.
34.
35.
36.
37.
38.
39.
40.
41.
42.

SECTION 10: BIRD EXTERNAL STRUCTURE

1. NAPE
2. CROWN
3. THROAT
4. MALAR
5. LESSER SECONDARY COVERTS
6. MEDIAN SECONDARY COVERTS
7. ALULA
8. GREATER SECONDARY COVERTS
9. PRIMARY COVERTS
10. MANTLE
11. SCAPULARS
12. TERTIALS
13. RUMP
14. UPPER TAIL COVERTS
15. TAIL
16. FOREHEAD
17. EYEBROW STRIPE
18. CROWN
19. EYE RING
20. EAR COVERTS
21. NAPE
22. BACK
23. UPPER MANDIBLE
24. NOSTRIL
25. LOWER MANDIBLE
26. LORE
27. BREAST
28. FLANK
29. TIBIA
30. TARSUS
31. FOOT
32. CLAW
33. RUMP
34. PRIMARY WING FEATHERS
35. UPPER TAIL COVERTS
36. UNDERTAIL COVERTS
37. TAIL
38. RACHIS
39. VANE
40. AFTERFEATHER
41. DOWNY BARBS
42. HOLLOW SHAFT

SECTION 11: RAT SKELETON AND INTERNAL STRUCTURE

1. _____
2. _____
3. _____
4. _____
5. _____
6. _____
7. _____
8. _____
9. _____
10. _____
11. _____
12. _____
13. _____
14. _____
15. _____
16. _____
17. _____
18. _____
19. _____

20. _____
21. _____
22. _____
23. _____
24. _____
25. _____
26. _____

27. _____
28. _____
29. _____
30. _____
31. _____
32. _____
33. _____
34. _____
35. _____
35. _____

27. _____
28. _____
29. _____
30. _____
31. _____
32. _____
33. _____
34. _____

SECTION 11: RAT SKELETON AND INTERNAL STRUCTURE

1. SUBMAXILLARY SALIVARY GLAND
2. LARYNX
3. THYROID GLAND
4. ESOPHAGUS
5. TRACHEA
6. THYMUS GLAND
7. HEART
8. LUNG
9. DIAPHRAGM
10. LIVER
11. STOMACH
12. DUODENUM
13. SPLEEN
14. PANCREAS
15. ILEUM
16. DESCENDING COLON
17. RECTUM
18. CECUM
19. ANUS
20. SKULL
21. ATLAS
22. AXIS
23. RIB
24. STERNUM
25. ILIUM
26. SACRUM
27. PATELLA
28. FEMUR
29. TIBIA
30. FIBULA
31. ISCHIUM
32. PUBIS
33. METATARSAL
34. TARSAL

SECTION 12: RAT MUSCLES AND EXTERNAL STRUCTURE

1.
2.
3.
4.
5.
6.
7.
8.
9.
10.
11.
12.
13.
14.
15.
16.
17.

SECTION 12: RAT MUSCLES AND EXTERNAL STRUCTURE

1. TEMPORALIS
2. MASSETER
3. STERNOMASTOIDEUS
4. CLAVOTRAPEZIUS
5. LEVATOR SCAPULAE VENTRALIS
6. ACROMIOTRAPEZIUS
7. SPINODELTOIDEUS
8. SPINOTRAPEZIUS
9. LATISSIMUS DORSI
10. TENSOR FASCIAE LATAE
11. GLUTEUS MAXIMUS
12. SEMITENDINOSUS
13. BICEPS FEMORIS
14. EXTERNAL OBLIQUE
15. TRICEPS
16. BRACHIALIS
17. BICEPS

SECTION 13: RABBIT SKELETON AND INTERNAL STRUCTURE

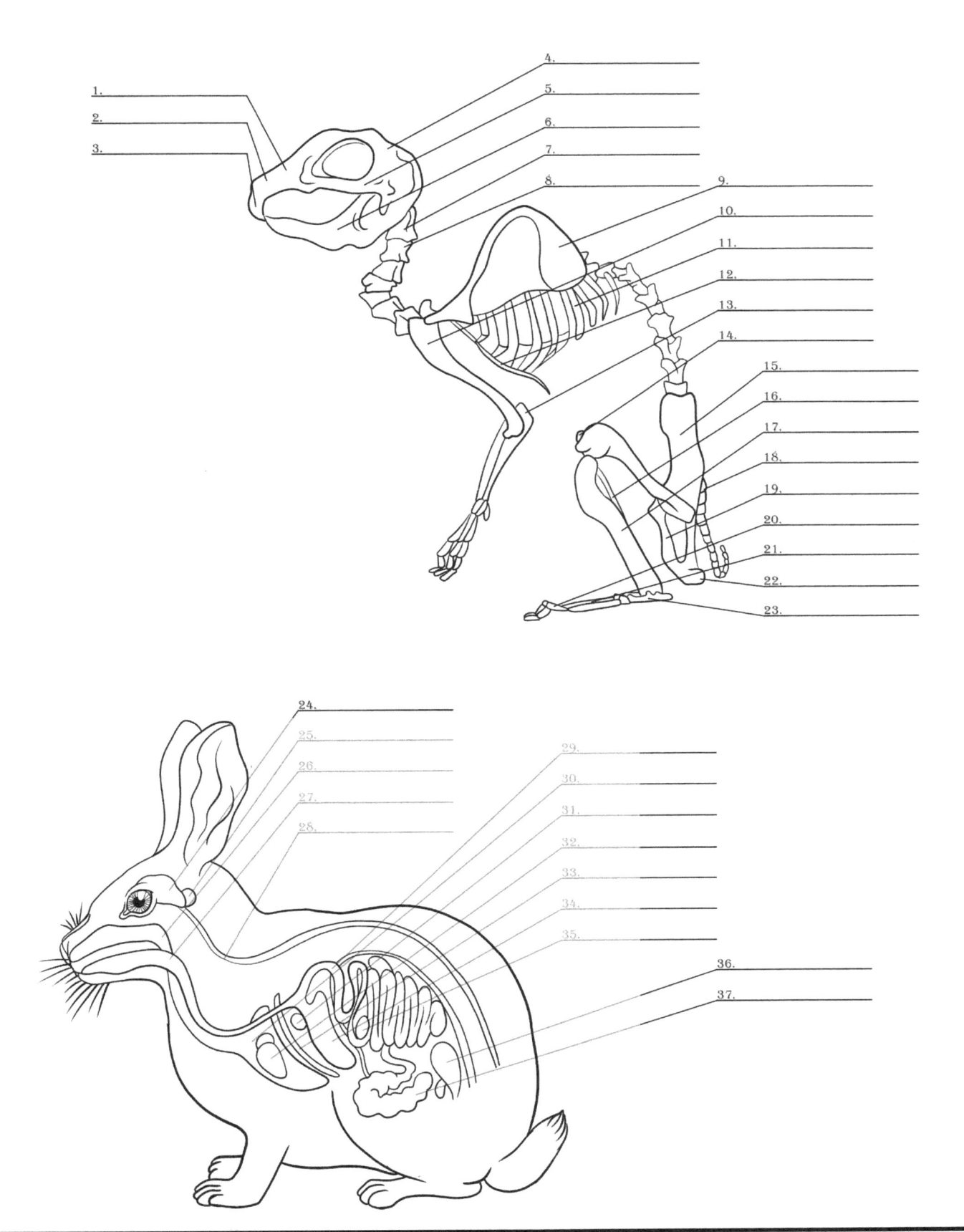

1.
2.
3.

4.
5.
6.
7.
8.
9.
10.
11.
12.
13.
14.
15.
16.
17.
18.
19.
20.
21.
22.
23.

24.
25.
26.
27.
28.

29.
30.
31.
32.
33.
34.
35.
36.
37.

SECTION 13: RABBIT SKELETON AND INTERNAL STRUCTURE

1. MAXILLA
2. NASAL
3. INCISOR
4. SKULL
5. ZYGOMATIC ARCH
6. MANDIBLE
7. ATLAS
8. AXIS
9. SCAPULA
10. HUMERUS
11. RIB
12. STERUM
13. ULNA
14. PATELLA
15. ILIUM
16. FIBULA
17. TIBIA
18. SACRUM
19. PUBIS
20. PHALANGE
21. METATARSAL
22. ISCHIUM
23. TARSAL
24. CEREBRUM
25. CEREBELLUM
26. TRACHEA
27. ESOPHAGUS
28. SPINAl CORD
29. LUNG
30. DUODENUM
31. GALL BLADDER
32. HEART
33. DIAPHRAGM
34. STOMACH
35. PANCREAS
36. BLADDER
37. CECUM

SECTION 14: RABBIT MUSCLES AND EXTERNAL STRUCTURE

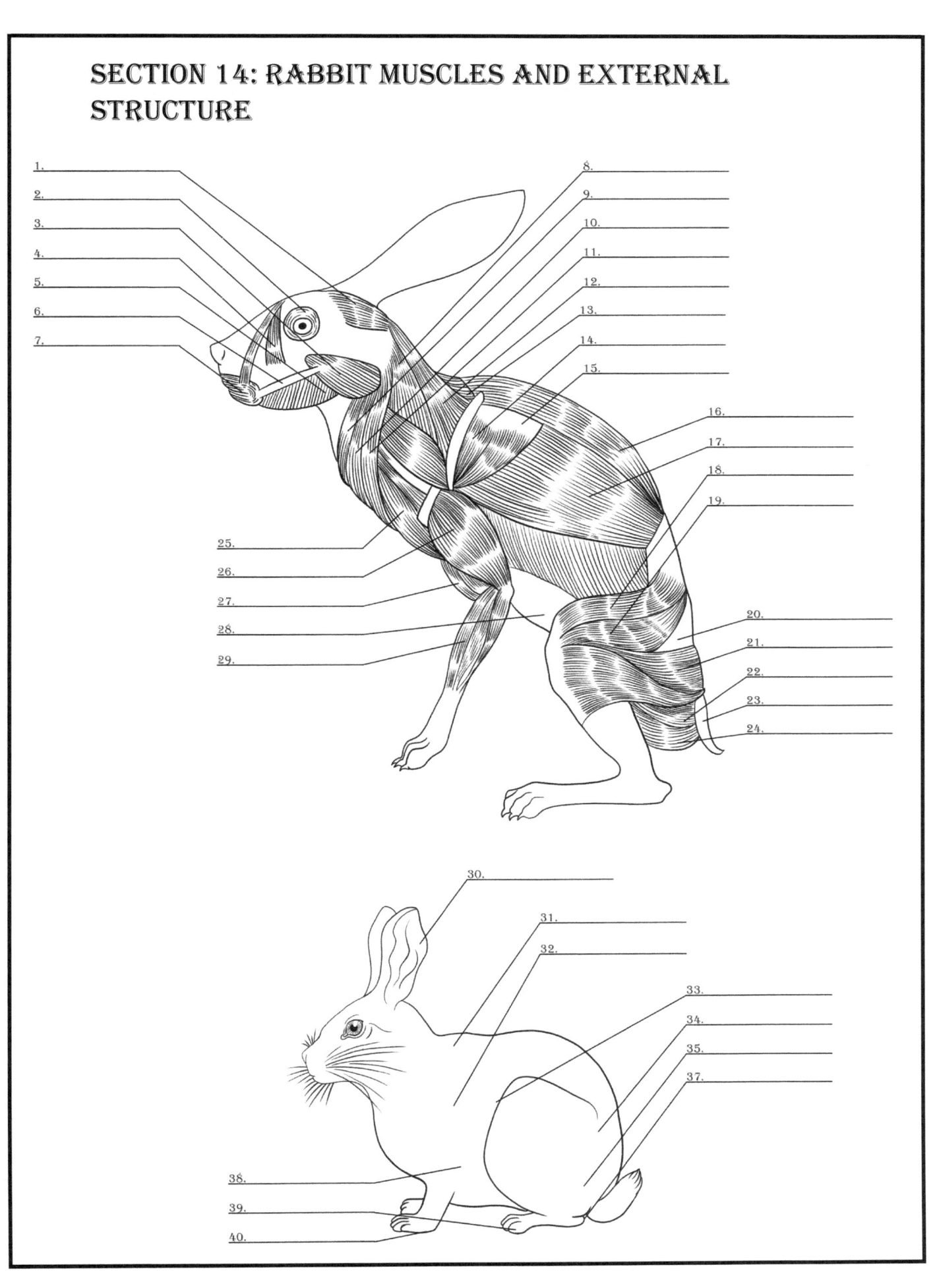

1. _____
2. _____
3. _____
4. _____
5. _____
6. _____
7. _____

8. _____
9. _____
10. _____
11. _____
12. _____
13. _____
14. _____
15. _____
16. _____
17. _____
18. _____
19. _____

20. _____
21. _____
22. _____
23. _____
24. _____

25. _____
26. _____
27. _____
28. _____
29. _____

30. _____
31. _____
32. _____
33. _____
34. _____
35. _____
37. _____

38. _____
39. _____
40. _____

SECTION 14: RABBIT MUSCLES AND EXTERNAL STRUCTURE

1. TEMPORALIS
2. ORBICULARIS OCULI
3. MASSETER
4. MALARIA
5. BUCCINATOR
6. ZYGOMATICUS
7. ORBICULARIS ORIS
8. SPLENIUS
9. STERNOHYOID
10. STERNOMASTOIDEUS
11. CLEIDOMASTOID
12. TRAPEZIUS
13. SUPRASPINATUS
14. DELTOID
15. INFRASPINATUSM
16. TRAPEZIUS
17. LATISSIMUS DORSI
18. TENSOR FASCIAE LATAE
19. RECTUS FEMORIS
20. GLUTEUS
21. BICEPS FEMORIS
22. SBMIMEMBRANOSUS
23. COCCYGEUS
24. SEMITENDINOSUS
25. BRACHIOCEPHALICUS
26. TRICEPS BRACHII
27. BRACHIALIS
28. RECTUS ABDOMINIS
29. EXTENSOR CARPI RADIALIS

SECTION 15: CANINE SKELETON AND INTERNAL STRUCTURE

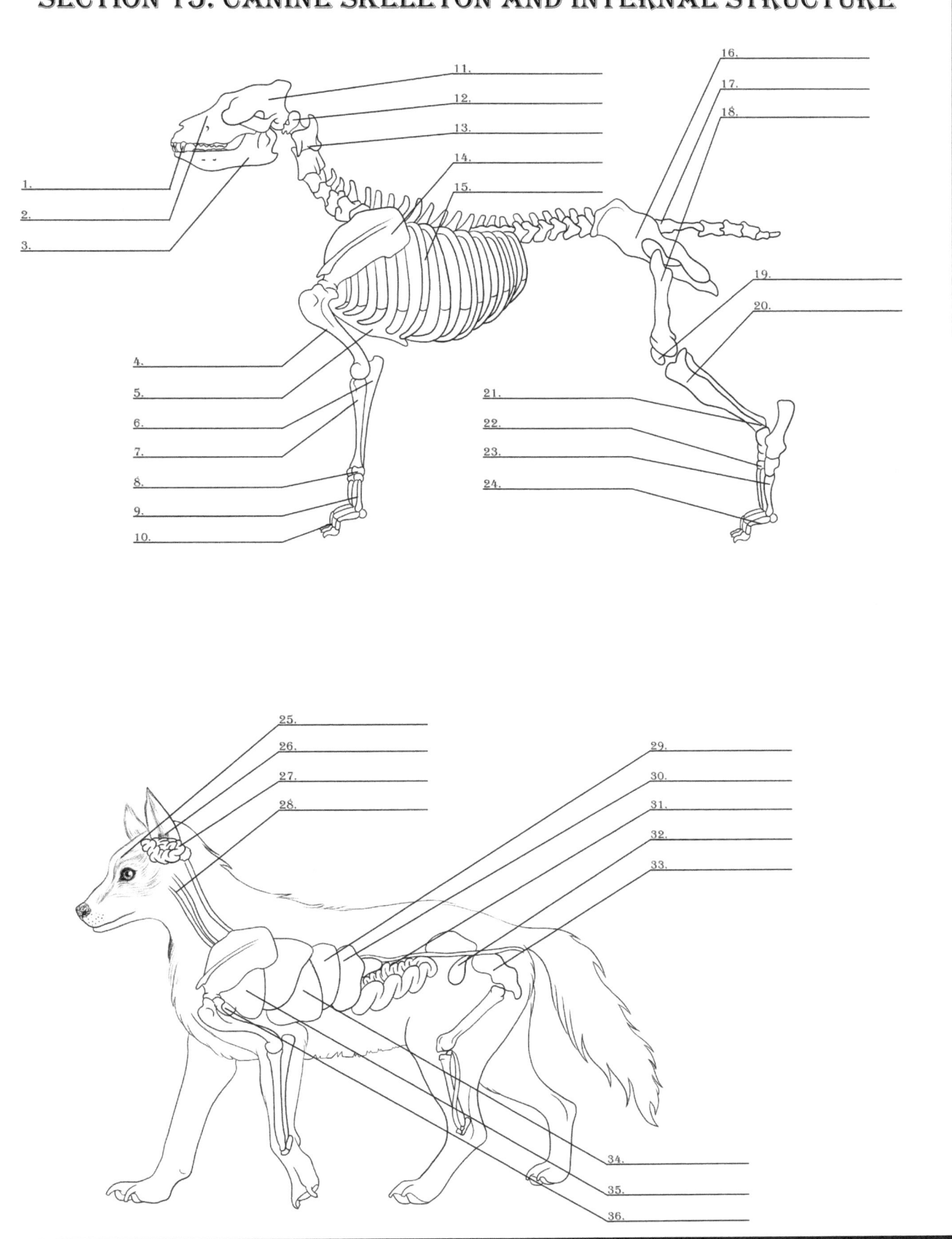

11.

12.

13.

14.

15.

16.

17.

18.

1.

2.

3.

19.

20.

4.

5.

6.

7.

8.

9.

10.

21.

22.

23.

24.

25.

26.

27.

28.

29.

30.

31.

32.

33.

34.

35.

36.

SECTION 15: CANINE SKELETON AND INTERNAL STRUCTURE

1. CANINE TOOTH
2. UPPER JAW
3. LOWER JAW
4. HUMERUS
5. STERNUM
6. ULNA
7. RADIUS
8. CARPUS
9. METACARPUS
10. CLAW
11. SKULL
12. ATLAS
13. AXIS
14. SCAPULA
15. RIB
16. PELVIS
17. SACRUM
18. FEMUR
19. PATELLA
20. TIBIA
21. FIBULA
22. TARSUS
23. METATARSUS
24. PHALANGE
25. NASAL CAVITY
26. CEREBRUM
27. CEREBELLUM
28. ESOPHAGUS
29. STOMACH
30. SPLEEN
31. INTESTINE
32. BLADDER
33. RECTUM
34. LIVER
35. LUNG
36. HEART

SECTION 16: CANINE MUSCLES

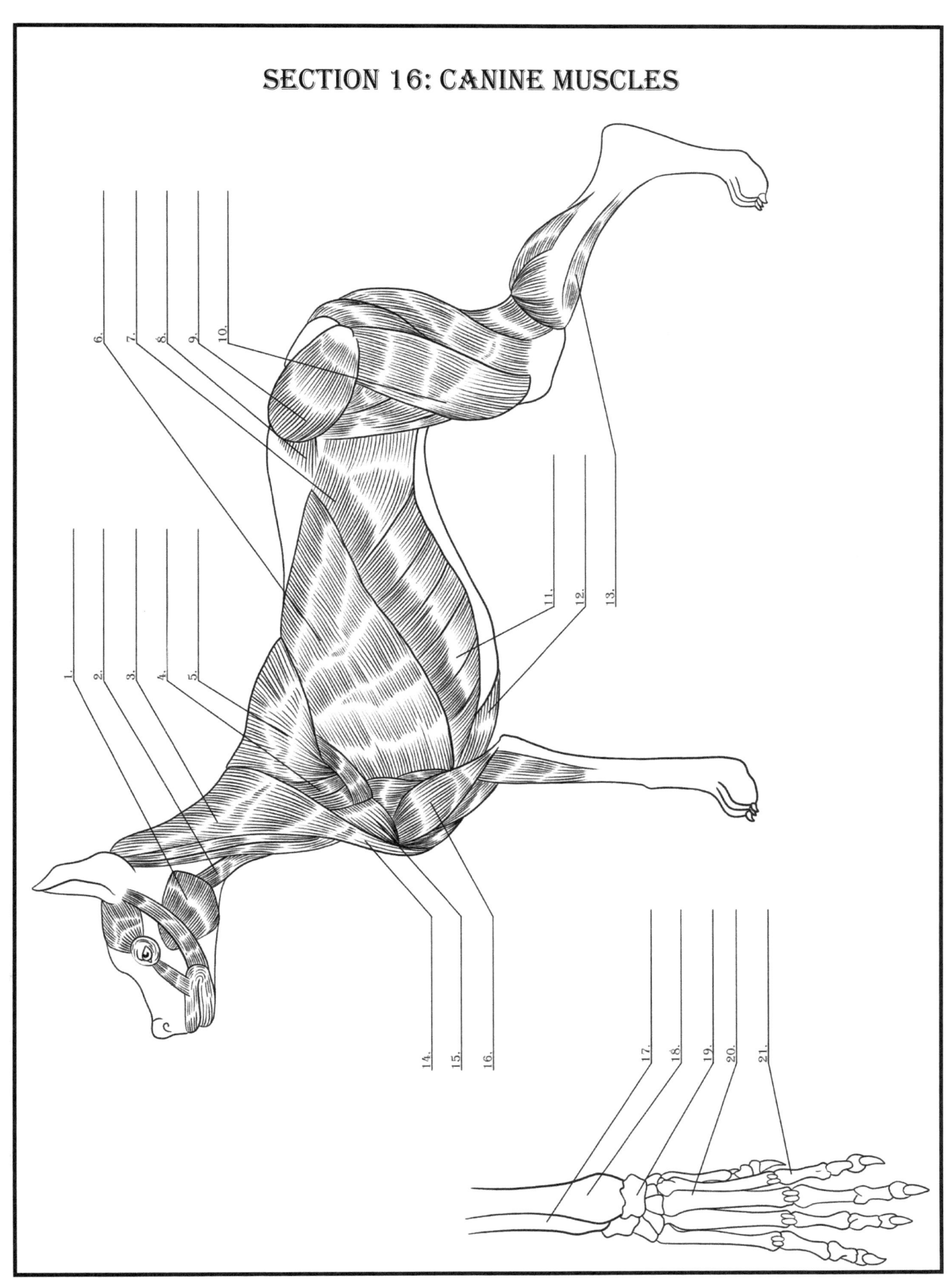

SECTION 16: CANINE MUSCLES

1. MASSETER
2. STERNOHYOID
3. BRACHIOCEPHALICUS
4. OMOTRANSVERSARIUS
5. TRAPEZIUS
6. LATISSIMUS DORSI
7. OBLIQUUS EXTERNUS ABDOMINIS
8. OBLIQUUS INTERNUS ABDOMINIS
9. GLUTEUS MEDIUS
10. BICEPS FEMORIS
11. INTERCOSTALIS EXTERNUS
12. PECTORALIS PROFUNDUS
13. CRANIAL TIBIAL
14. CLAVICULAR TENDINOUS SEPTUM
15. DELTOIDEUS
16. TRICEPS BRACHII
17. ULNA
18. RADIUS
19. CARPAL
20. METACARPAL
21. DIGIT

SECTION 17: FELINE SKELETON AND INTERNAL STRUCTURE

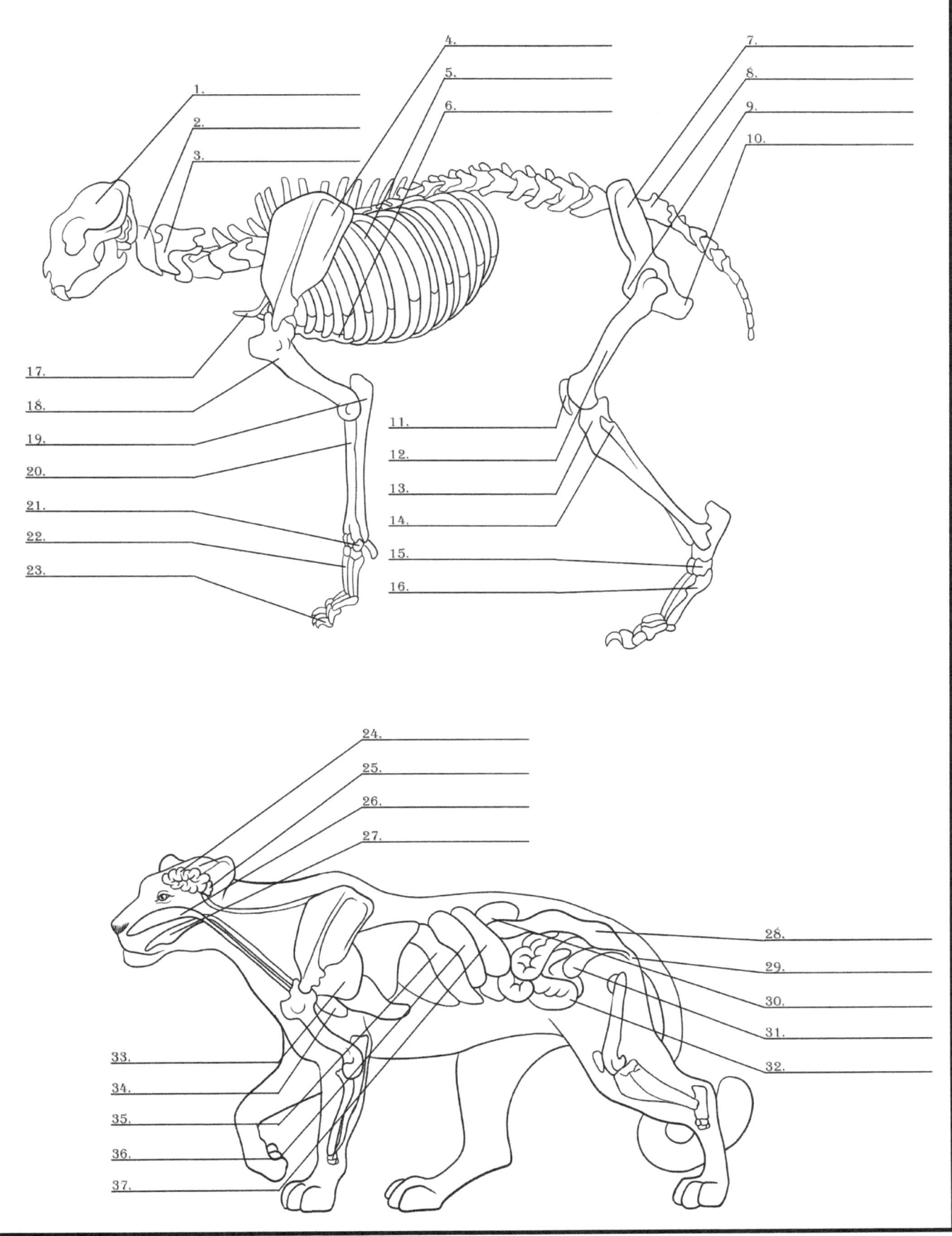

1.

2.

3.

4.

5.

6.

7.

8.

9.

10.

11.

12.

13.

14.

15.

16.

17.

18.

19.

20.

21.

22.

23.

24.

25.

26.

27.

28.

29.

30.

31.

32.

33.

34.

35.

36.

37.

SECTION 17: FELINE SKELETON AND INTERNAL STRUCTURE

1. SKULL
2. ATLAS
3. AXIS
4. SCAPULA
5. RIB
6. STERNUM
7. HIP BONE
8. SACRUM
9. PUBIC BONE
10. ISCHIAL BONE
11. PATELLA
12. FEMUR
13. TIBIA
14. FIBULA
15. TARSAL
16. METATARSAK
17. CLAVICLE
18. HUMERUS
19. ULNA
20. RADIUS
21. CARPAL
22. METACARPAL
23. CLAW
24. CEREBRUM
25. CEREBELLUM
26. NASAL CAVITY
27. TONGUE
28. COLON
29. ANUS
30. BLADDER
31. KIDNEY
32. SMALL INTESTINE
33. LUNG
34. HEART
35. LIVER
36. STOMACH
37. SPLEEN

SECTION 18: FELINE MUSCLES

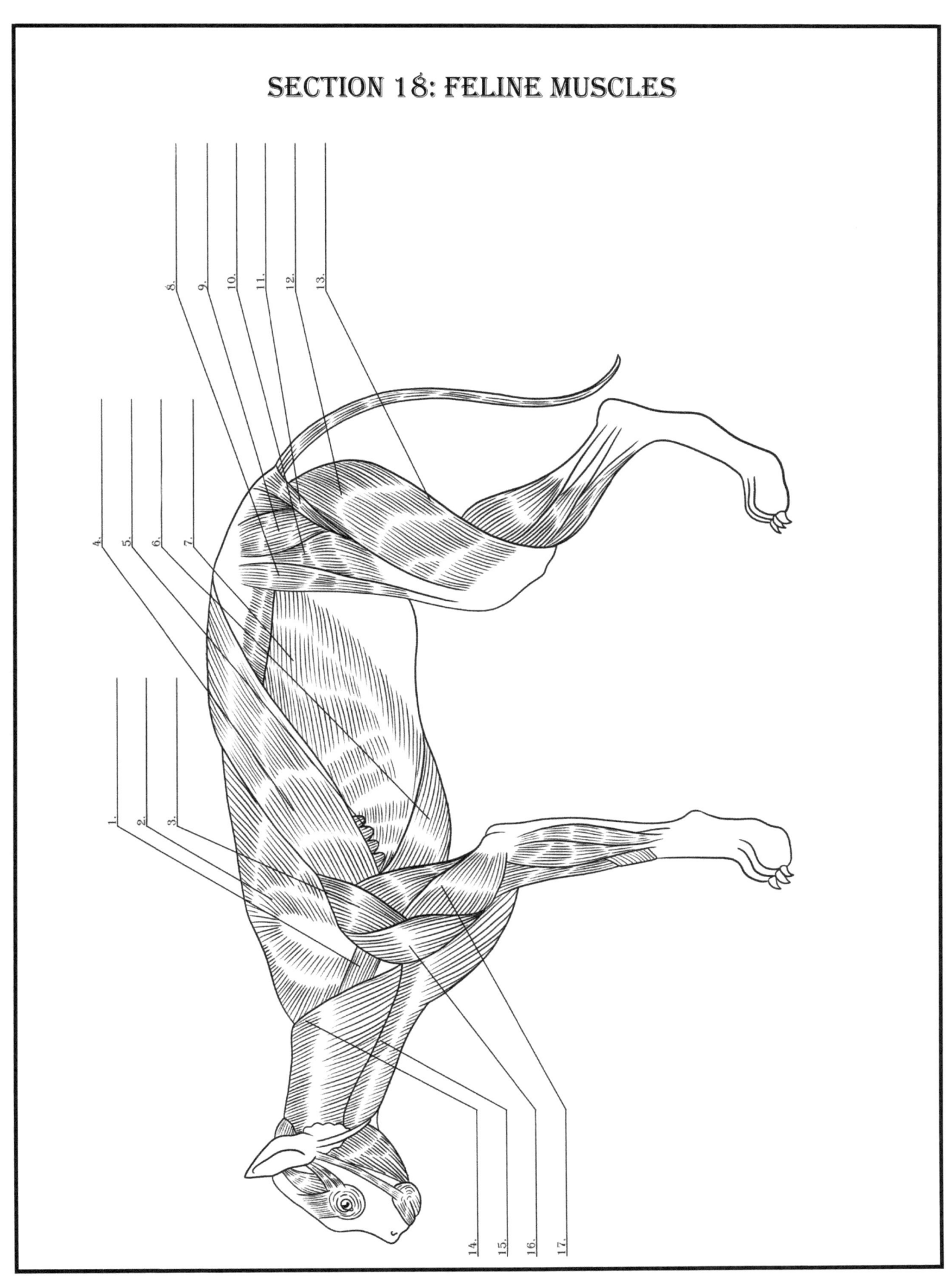

SECTION 18: FELINE MUSCLES

1. OMOTRANSVERSARIUS
2. TRAPEZIUS
3. INFRASPINATUS
4. LATISSIMUS DORSI
5. SERRATUS VENTRALIS
6. PECTORALIS PROFUNDUS
7. EXTERNAL OBLIQUE ABDOMINAL
8. SARTORIUS
9. GLUTEUS MEDIUS
10. TENSOR FASCIAE LATAE
11. CAUDOFEMORALIS
12. BICEPS FEMORIS
13. SEMITENDINOSUS
14. BRACHIOCEPHALICUS
15. STERNOCEPHALICUS
16. DELTOIDEUS
17. TRICEPS BRACHII

SECTION 19: SHEEP SKELETON AND INTERNAL STRUCTURE

1. _____

2. _____

3. _____

4. _____

5. _____

6. _____

7. _____

8. _____

9. _____

10. _____

11. _____

12. _____

13. _____

14. _____

15. _____

16. _____

17. _____

18. _____

19. _____

20. _____

21. _____

22. _____

23. _____

24. _____

25. _____

26. _____

27. _____

28. _____

SECTION 19: SHEEP SKELETON AND INTERNAL STRUCTURE

1. ATLAS
2. ORBIT
3. AXIS
4. MAXILLA
5. MANDIBLE
6. SCAPULA
7. HUMERUS
8. RIB
9. STERNUM
10. RADIUS
11. ULNA
12. ISCHIAL TUBER
13. PELVIS
14. HIP JOINT
15. COSTAL ARCH, THE KNEE OF THE RIB
16. TIBIA
17. CEREBRUM
18. CEREBELLUM
19. TRACHEA
20. ESOPHAGUS
21. SPINAL CORD
22. ABOMASUM
23. DORSAL SAC OF RUMEN
24. VENTRAL SAC OF RUMEN
25. SMALL INTESTINE
26. LUNG
27. SPLEEN
28. HEART

SECTION 20: SHEEP MUSCLES

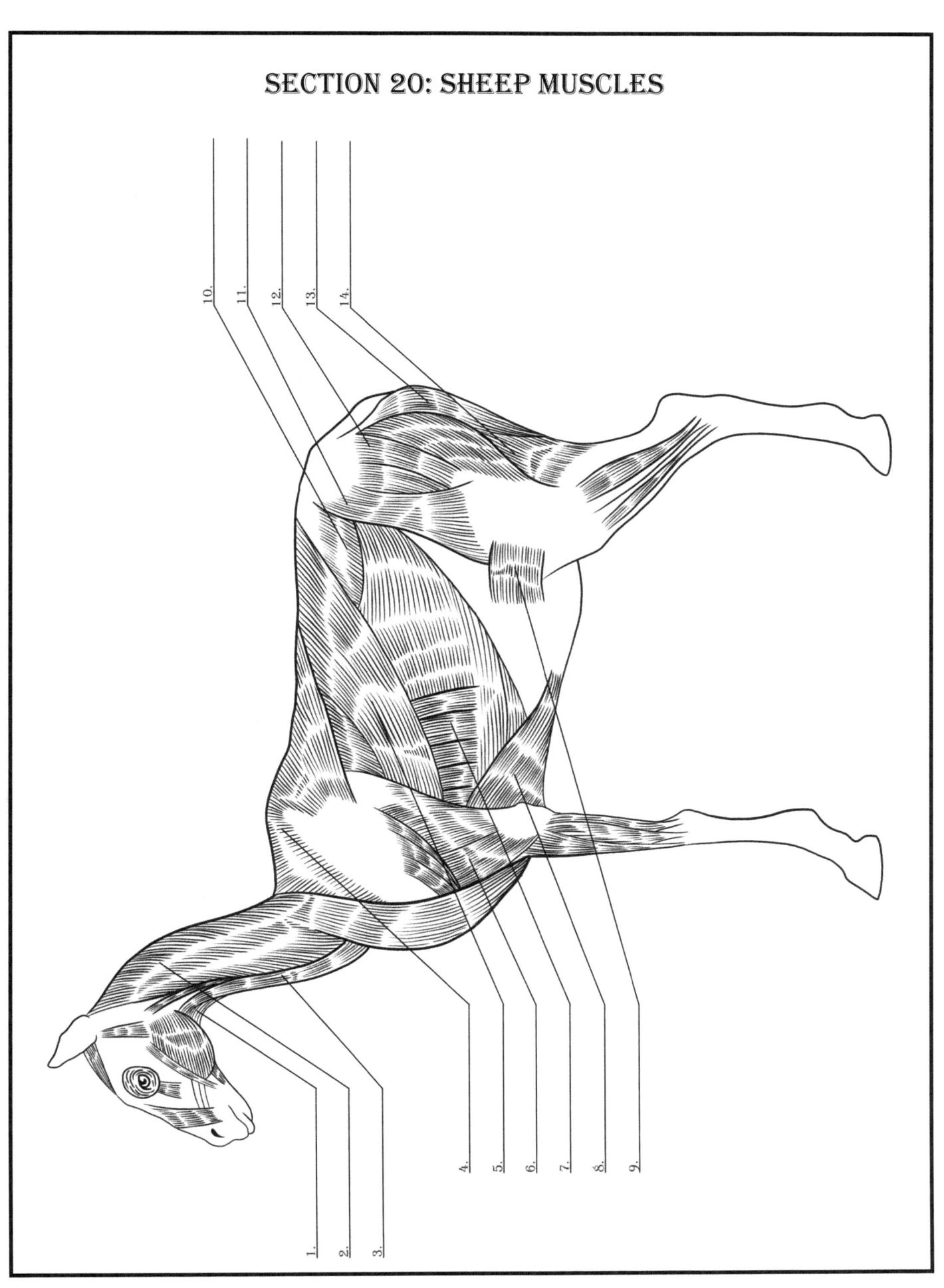

SECTION 20: SHEEP MUSCLES

1. STERNOHYOIDEUS
2. BRACHIOCEPHALICUS
3. STERNOCEPHALICUS
4. TRAPEZIUS
5. LATISSIMUS DORSI
6. TRICEPS BRACHII
7. SERRATUS VENTRALIS
8. PECTORALIS PROFUNDUS
9. CUTANEUS PLICAE
10. OBLIQUUS INTERNUS ABDOMINIS
11. TENSOR FASCIAE LATAE
12. GLUTEUS PROXIMALIS
13. SEMITENDINOSUS
14. GLUTEOBICEPS

SECTION 21: PIG SKELETON AND INTERNAL STRUCTURE

1. _____
2. _____
3. _____
4. _____
5. _____

6. _____
7. _____
8. _____

9. _____
10. _____
11. _____
12. _____
13. _____
14. _____
15. _____
16. _____
17. _____

18. _____
19. _____
20. _____

21. _____
22. _____
23. _____
24. _____

25. _____
26. _____
27. _____
28. _____

29. _____
30. _____
31. _____
32. _____
33. _____

SECTION 21: PIG SKELETON AND INTERNAL STRUCTURE

1. SKULL
2. OCCIPITAL CREST
3. MAXILLA
4. ATLAS
5. AXIS
6. PELVIS
7. SACRUM
8. FEMUR
9. MANDIBLE
10. SCAPULA
11. HUMERUS
12. RIB
13. STERNUM
14. RADIUS
15. ULNA
16. CARPAL
17. METACARPAL
18. PATELLA
19. TIBIA
20. FIBULA
21. CEREBRUM
22. CEREBELLUM
23. SPINAL CORD
24. TRACHEA
25. KIDNEY
26. SPLEEN
27. RECTUM
28. SMALL INTESTINE
29. LUNG
30. HEART
31. STOMACH
32. LIVER
33. BLADDER

SECTION 22: PIG MUSCLES

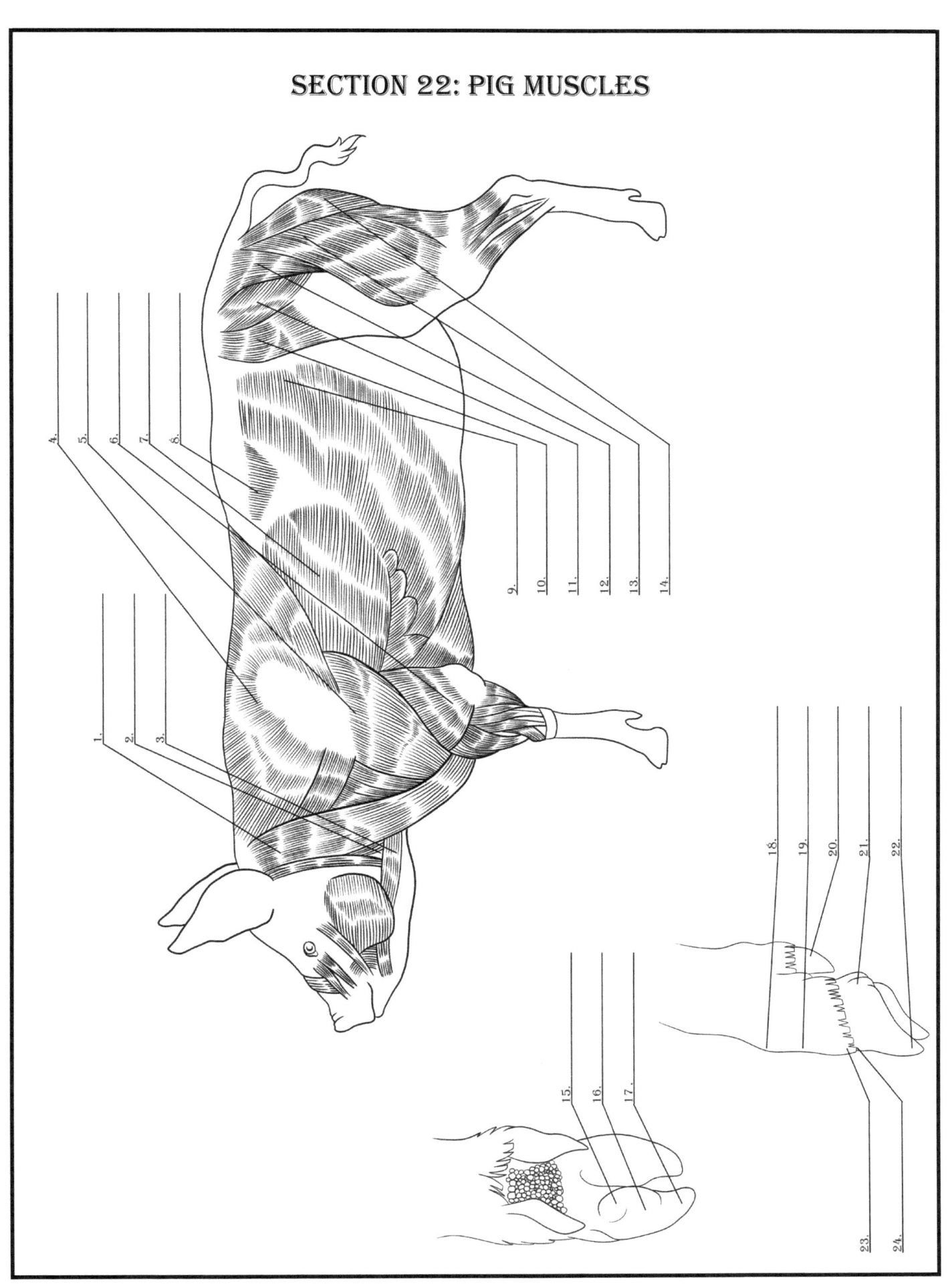

SECTION 22: PIG MUSCLES

1. BRACHIOCEPHALICUS
2. PAROTIDEOAURICULARIS
3. STERNOHYOIDEUS
4. TRAPEZIUS
5. DELTOIDEUS
6. TRICEPS BRACHII
7. LATISSIMUS DORSI
8. SERRATUS DORSALIS
9. OBLIQUUS EXTERNUS ABDOMINIS
10. TENSOR FASCIAE LATAE
11. GLUTEUS MEDIUS
12. GLUTEUS SUPERFICIALIS
13. BICEPS FEMORIS
14. SEMITENDINOSUS
15. DIGITAL CUSHION
16. SOLE
17. BORDER OF THE SOLE
18. REGION OF THE FETLOCK JOINTS
19. REGION OF THE PASTERN JOINTS
20. DEWCLAW
21. PALMAR/PLANTAR BORDER OF THE HORNY WALL
22. THE TIP OF THE HORNY WALL
23. PERIOPLE
24. CORONET REGION

SECTION 23: HORSE SKELETON AND INTERNAL STRUCTURE

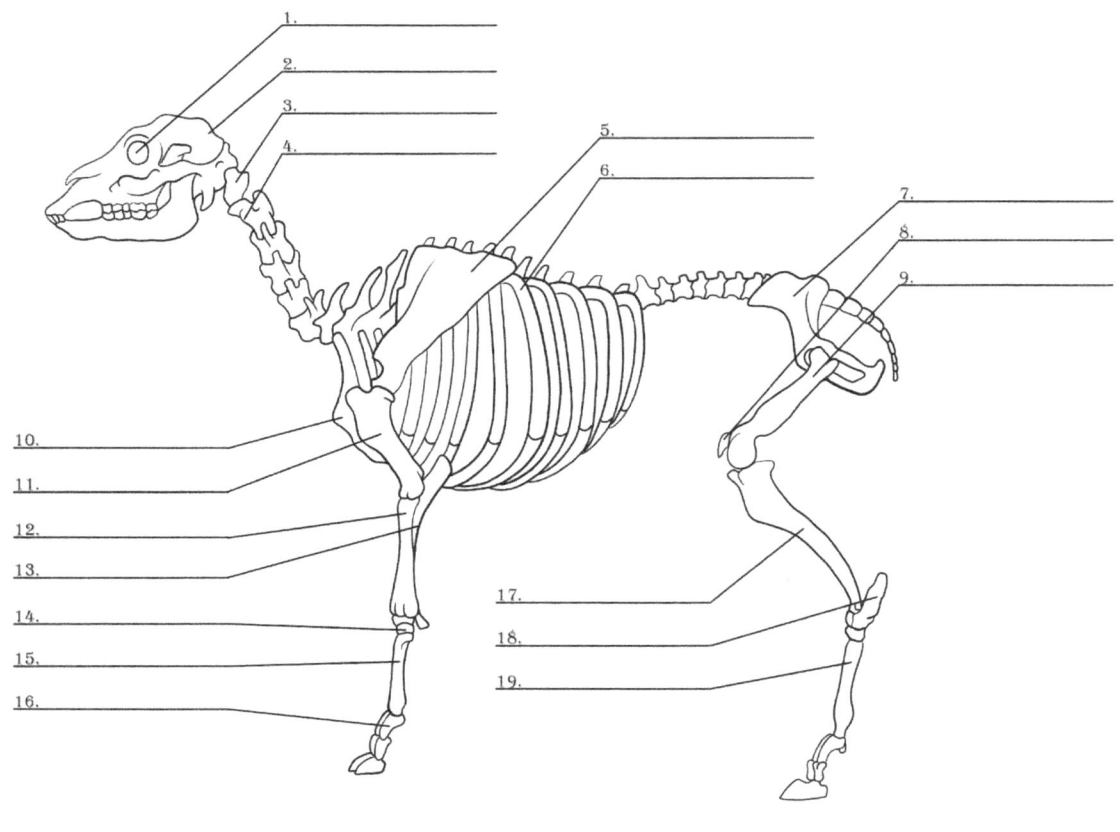

1. _____
2. _____
3. _____
4. _____
5. _____
6. _____
7. _____
8. _____
9. _____
10. _____
11. _____
12. _____
13. _____
14. _____
15. _____
16. _____
17. _____
18. _____
19. _____

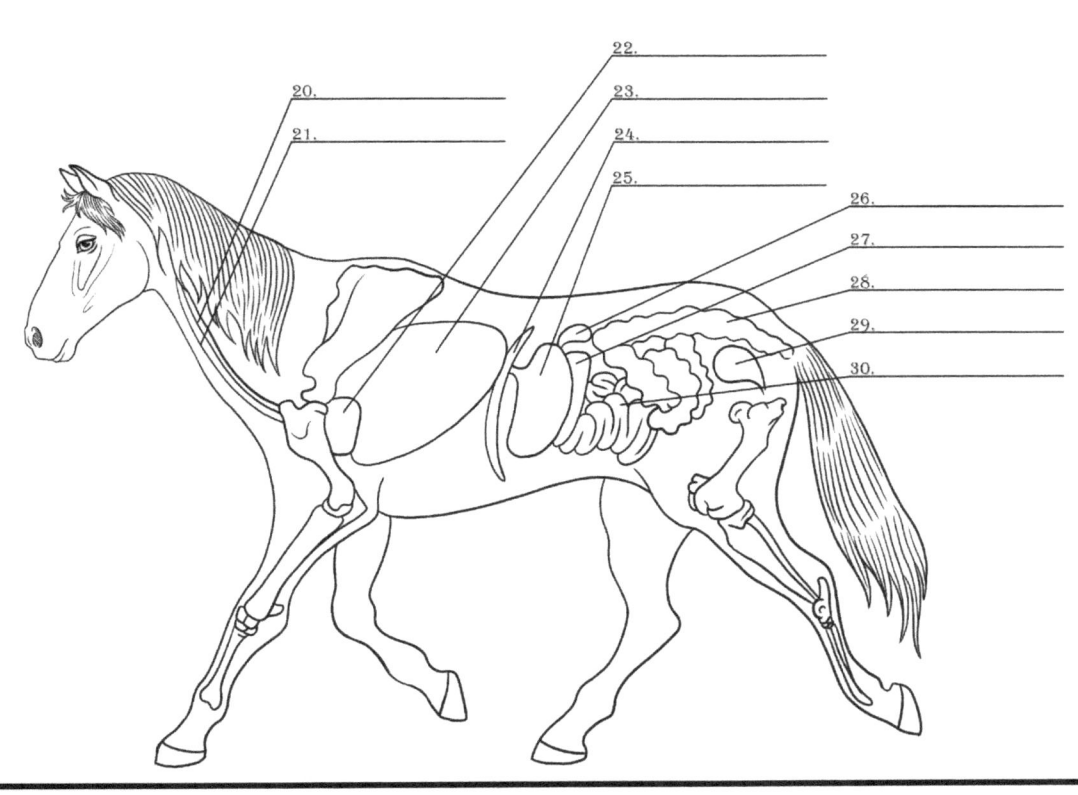

20. _____
21. _____
22. _____
23. _____
24. _____
25. _____
26. _____
27. _____
28. _____
29. _____
30. _____

SECTION 23: HORSE SKELETON AND INTERNAL STRUCTURE

1. ORBIT
2. SKULL
3. ATLAS
4. AXIS
5. SCAPULA
6. RIB
7. PELVIS
8. PATELLA
9. FEMUR
10. STERNUM
11. HUMERUS
12. RADIUS
13. ULNA
14. CARPAL
15. METACARPAL
16. PHALANGE
17. TIBIA
18. CALCANEOUS
19. METATARSAL
20. TRACHEA
21. ESOPHAGUS
22. HEART
23. LUNG
24. DIAPHRAGM
25. STOMACH
26. KIDNEY
27. SPLEEN
28. RECTUM
29. BLADDER
30. SMALL INTESTINE

SECTION 24: HORSE MUSCLES

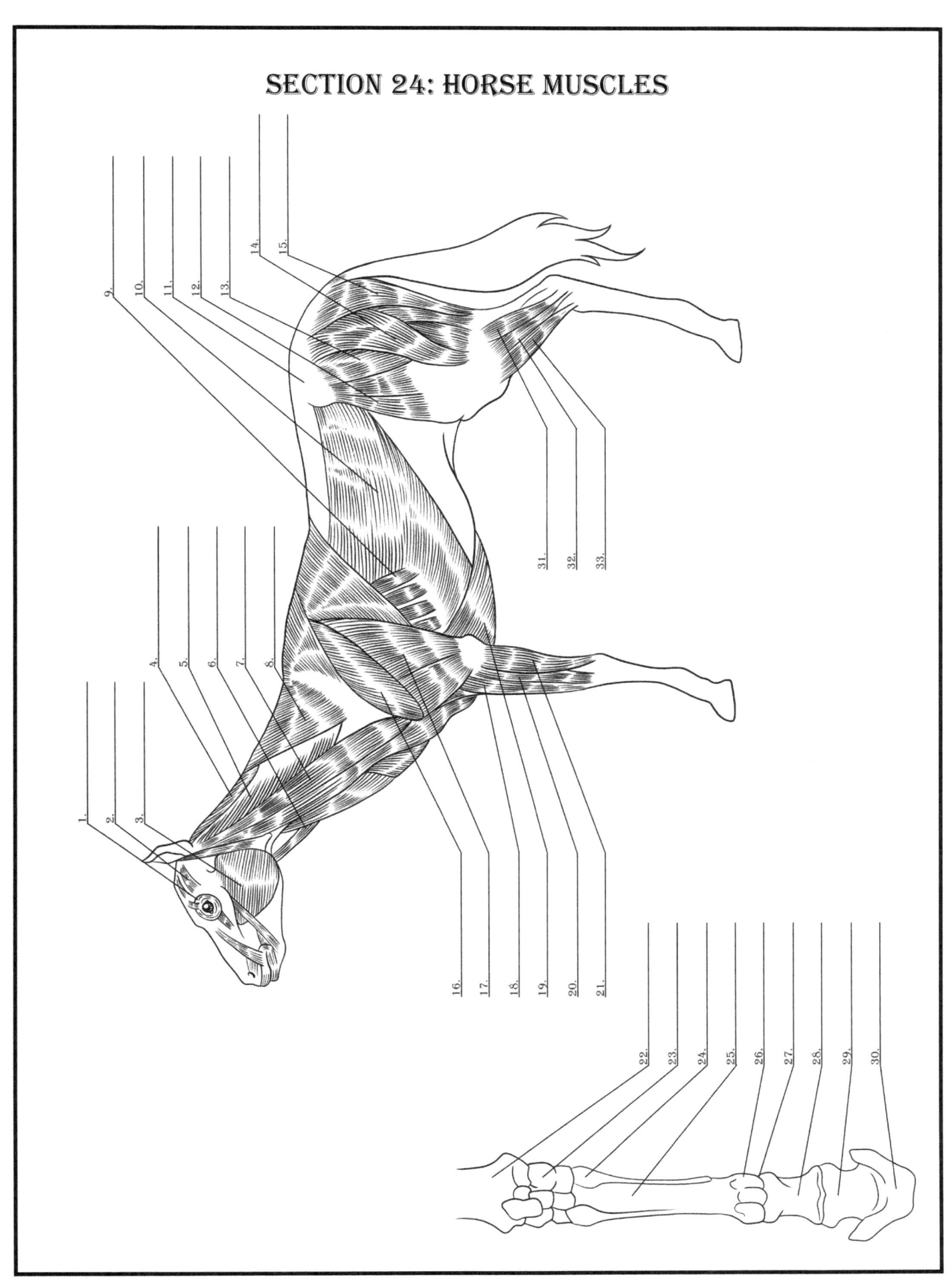

SECTION 24: HORSE MUSCLES

1. ORBICULARIS OCULI
2. TEMPORALIS
3. MASSETER
4. CERVICAL RHOMBOIDEUS
5. SPLENIUS
6. STERNOCEPHALICUS
7. BRACHIOCEPHALICUS
8. TRAPEZIUS
9. EXTERNAL INTERCOSTAL
10. EXTERNAL ABDOMINAL OBLIQUE
11. GLUTEAL FASCIA
12. TENSOR FASCIAE LATAE
13. GLUTEUS SUPERFICIALIS
14. BICEPS FEMORIS
15. SEMITENDINOSUS
16. DELTOIDEUS
17. TRICEPS BRACHII
18. EXTENSOR CARPI RADIALIS
19. PECTORALIS
20. TRICEPS
21. EXTENSOR CARPI ULNARIS
22. RADIUS
23. CARPUS
24. SPLINT BONE
25. METACARPAL (CANNON BONE)
26. PROXIMAL SESAMOIDS
27. METACARPAL-PHALANGAL (FETLOCK) JOINT
28. PROXIMAL PHALANX
29. MIDDLE PHALANX
30. DISTAL PHALANX
31. FLEXOR DIGITORUM PROFUNDUS
32. EXTENSOR DIGITORUM LATERALIS
33. EXTENSOR DIGITORUM LONGUS

SECTION 25: COW SKELETON AND INTERNAL STRUCTURE

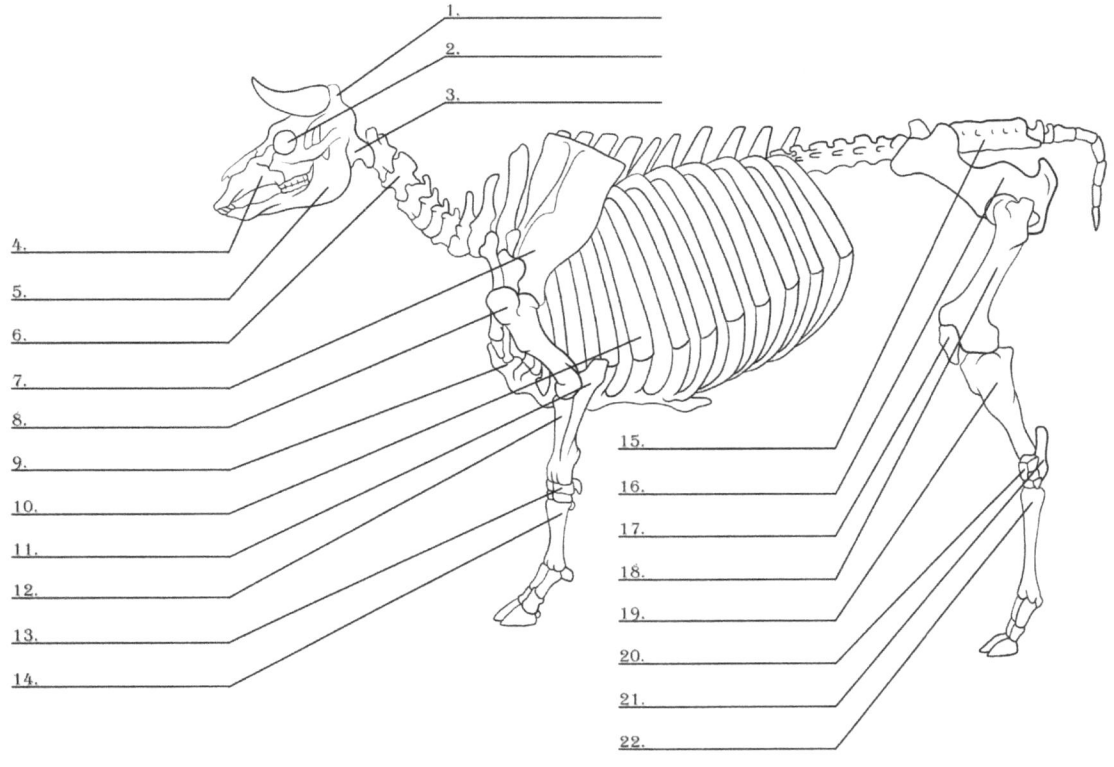

1. _____
2. _____
3. _____
4. _____
5. _____
6. _____
7. _____
8. _____
9. _____
10. _____
11. _____
12. _____
13. _____
14. _____

15. _____
16. _____
17. _____
18. _____
19. _____
20. _____
21. _____
22. _____

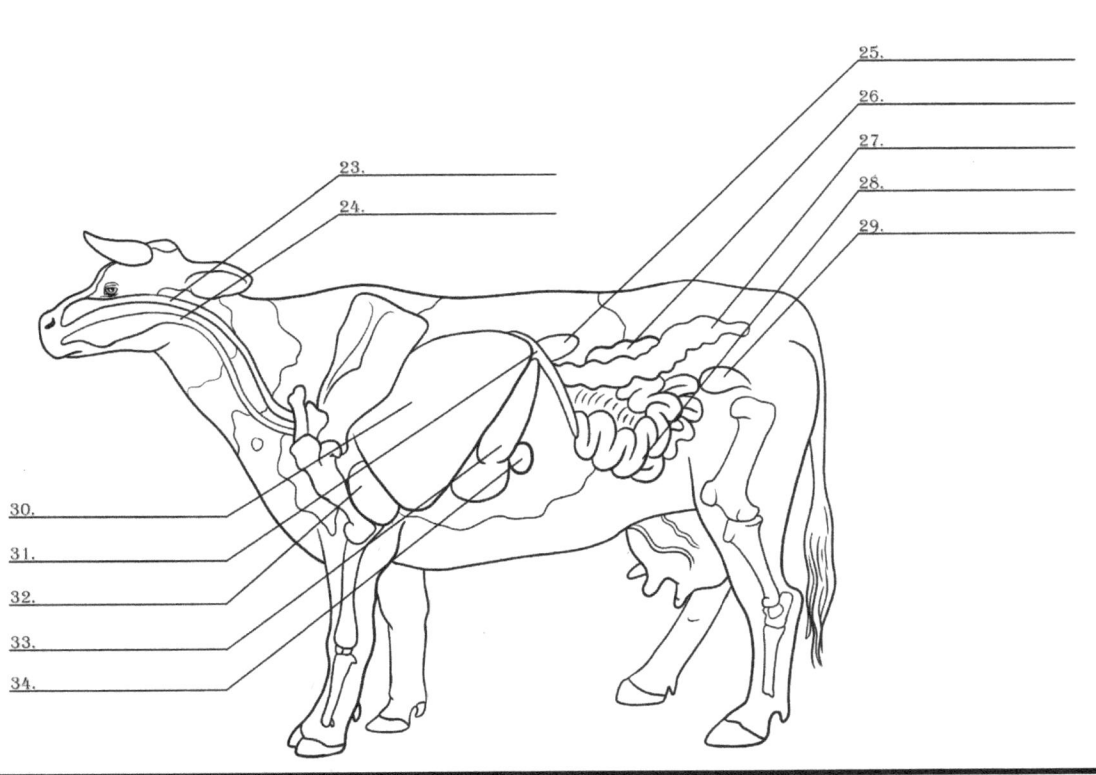

23. _____
24. _____

25. _____
26. _____
27. _____
28. _____
29. _____

30. _____
31. _____
32. _____
33. _____
34. _____

SECTION 25: COW SKELETON AND INTERNAL STRUCTURE

1. CORNUAL PROCESS OF THE FRONTAL BONE
2. ORBIT
3. ATLAS
4. MAXILLA
5. MANDIBLE
6. AXIS
7. SCAPULA
8. HUMERUS
9. STERNUM
10. RIB
11. ULNA
12. RADIUS
13. CARPUS
14. METACARPUS
15. SACRUM
16. PELVIS
17. PATELLA
18. FEMUR
19. TIBIA
20. TARSAL
21. CALCANEAL TTUBEROSITY
22. METATARSUS
23. TRACHEA
24. ESOPHAGUS
25. KIDNEY
26. DUODENUM
27. CECUM
28. JEJUNUM
29. BLADDER
30. LUNG
31. DIAPHRAGM
32. HEART
33. LIVER
34. GALL BLADDER

SECTION 26: COW MUSCLES

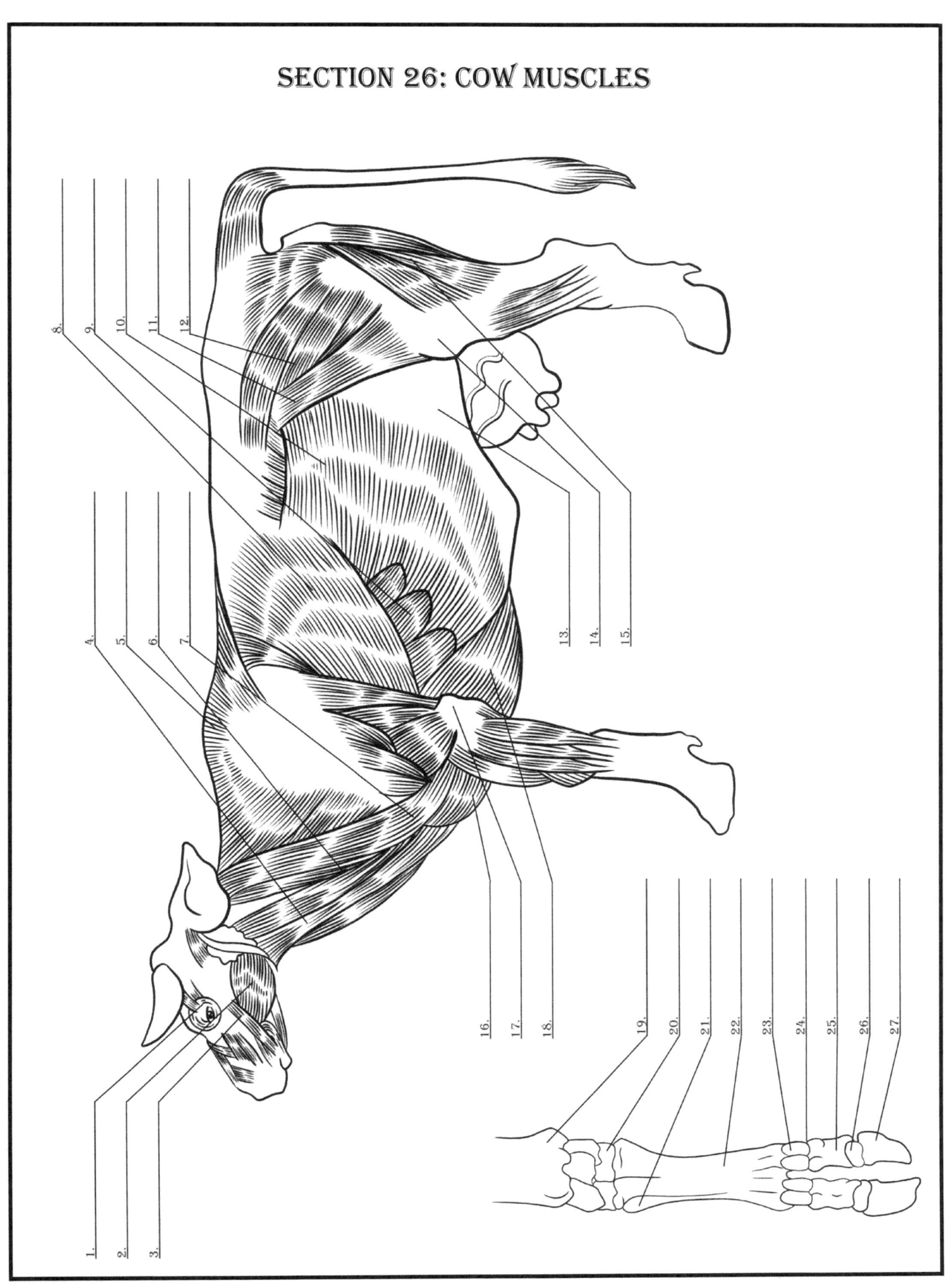

SECTION 26: COW MUSCLES

1. ORBICULARIS OCULI
2. MASSETER
3. ZYGOMATIC
4. STERNOMANDIBULARIS
5. TRAPEZIUS
6. CLEIDOMASTOIDEUS
7. BRACHIOCEPHALICUS
8. GLUTEUS PROXIMAL
9. SERRATUS VENTRALIS
10. OBLIQUUS EXTERNUS ABDOMINIS
11. TENSOR FASCIAE LATAE
12. GLUTEUS PROXIMALIS
13. YELLOW ABDOMINAL FASCIA (TUNICA FLAVA ABDOMINIS)
14. STIFLE JOINT
15. GLUTEUS CAUDALIS
16. PECTORALIS
17. TUBER OLECRANI WITH THE TRICEPS BRACHII MUSCLE
18. PECTORALIS
19. RADIUS
20. CARPUS
21. SPLINT BONE
22. METACARPAL (CANNON) BONE
23. PROXIMAL SESAMOIDS
24. METACARPAL-PHALANGAL (FETLOCK) JOINT
25. PROXIMAL PHALANX
26. MIDDLE PHALANX
27. DISTAL PHALANX

SECTION 27: ELEPHANT SKELETON AND INTERNAL STRUCTURE

1.
2.
3.
4.
5.
6.
7.
8.
9.
10.
11.
12.
13.
14.
15.
16.
17.
18.
19.
20.
21.
22.
23.
24.
25.
26.
27.
28.
29.
30.
31.
32.
33.
34.
35.
36.
37.
38.
39.
40.
41.
42.
43.
44.
45.
46.
47.

SECTION 27: ELEPHANT SKELETON AND INTERNAL STRUCTURE

1. SKULL
2. ROSTRAL BONE
3. TEMPORAL FOSSA
4. ORBITAL RIDGE
5. INCISOR (TRUNK SUPPORT)
6. SCAPULA
7. SCAPULAR SPINE
8. RIB
9. MANDIBLE
10. ZYGOMATIC ARCH
11. EAR OPENING
12. HUMERUS
13. STERNUM
14. OLECRANON
15. RADIUS
16. ULNA
17. CARPAL
18. METACARPAL
19. PHALANGE
20. PELVIS
21. SACRUM
22. FEMUR
23. PATELLA
24. TIBIA
25. FIBULA
26. CALCANEUS
27. TARSAL
28. METATARSAL
29. EAR
30. BRAIN
31. TONGUE
32. TRUNK
33. HEART
34. LUNG
35. DIAPHRAGM
36. SPINAL CORD
37. ESOPHAGUS
38. TRACHEA
39. KIDNEY
40. URETER
41. BLADDER
42. DUODENUM
43. SMALL INTESTINE
44. CECUM
45. ANUS
46. SPLEEN
47. STOMACH

SECTION 28: ELEPHANT MUSCLES

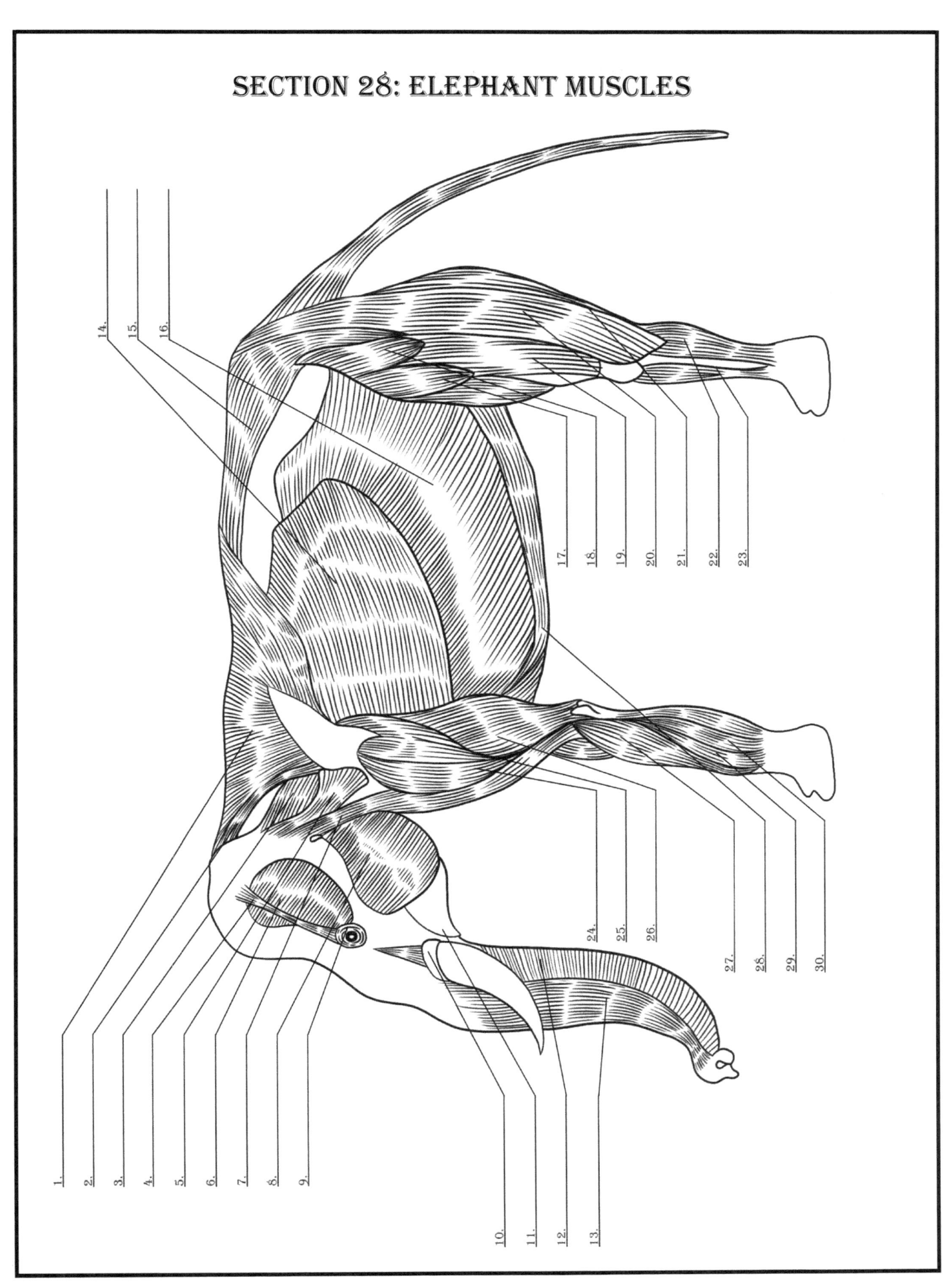

SECTION 28: ELEPHANT MUSCLES

1. TRAPEZIUS
2. RHOMBOID
3. SPLENIUS
4. OCCIPITO-FRONTALIS
5. OMOTRANSVERSARIUS
6. TEMPORALIS
7. BRACHIOCEPHALICUS
8. MASSETER
9. ORBICULARIS OCULI
10. BUCCINATOR, PARS SUPRALABIALIS
11. ORBICULARIS ORIS
12. BUCCINATOR, PARS RIMANA
13. LEVATOR LABII MAXILLARIS
14. LATISSIMUS DORSI
15. LONGISSIMUS DORSI
16. EXTERNAL ABDOMINAL OBLIQUE
17. TENSOR FASCIAE LATAE
18. GLUTEUS MEDICUS
19. GLUTEUS SUPERFICIAL
20. BICEPS FEMORIS
21. SEMITENDINOSUS
22. EXTENSOR LATERALIS
23. TIBIALIS CRANIALIS
24. DELTOID, ACROMIAL PORTION
25. DELTOID, SCAPULAR PORTION
26. TRICEPS
27. BRACHIORADIALIS
28. RECTUS ABDOMINALIS
29. EXTENSOR DIGITORUM COMMUNIS
30. ULNARIS

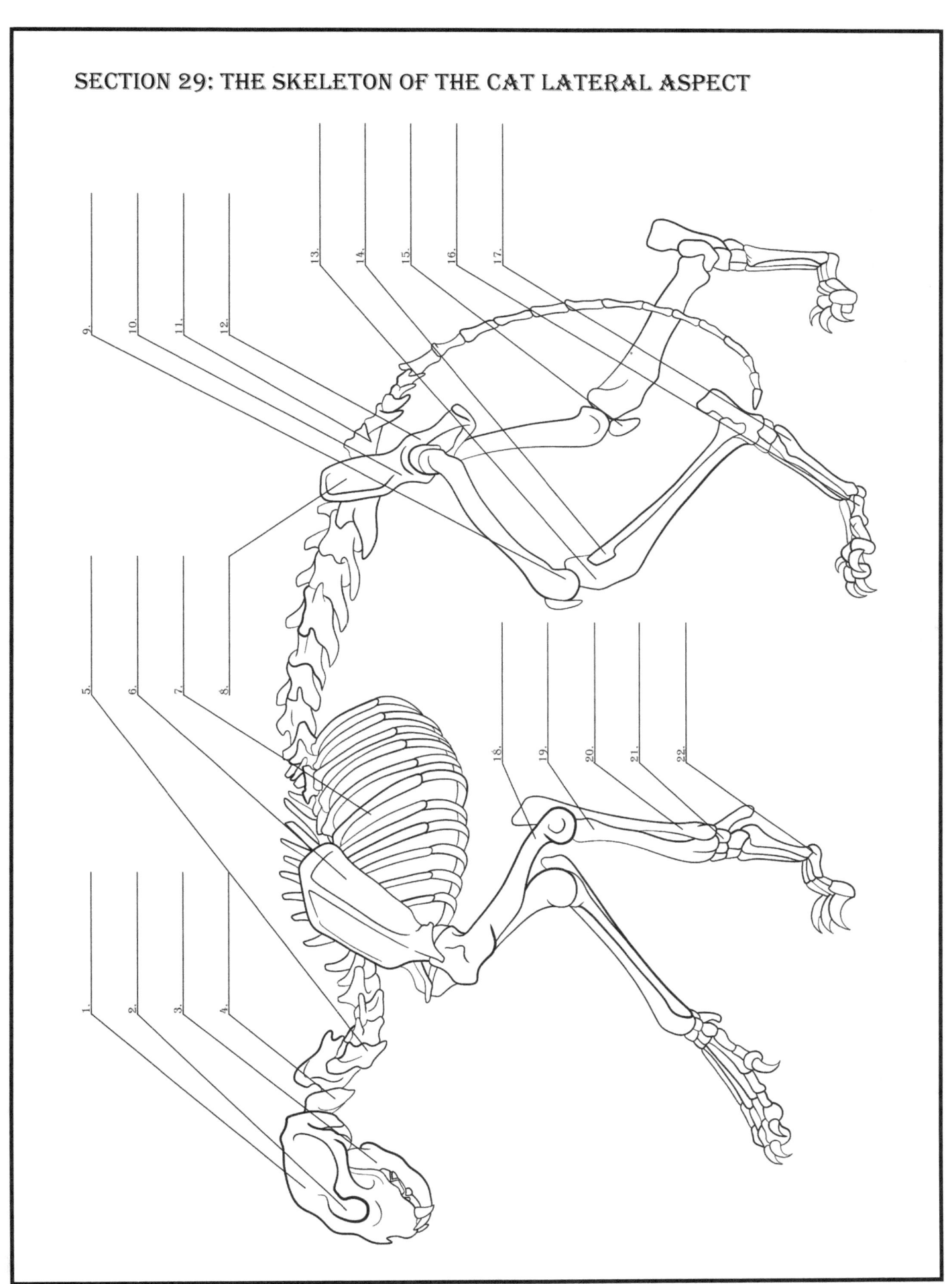

SECTION 29: THE SKELETON OF THE CAT LATERAL ASPECT

1. SKULL
2. ORBIT
3. MANDIBLE
4. ATLAS
5. AXIS
6. SCAPULA
7. RIB
8. ILIUM
9. FEMUR
10. PUBIS
11. SACRUM
12. ISCHIUM
13. TIBIA
14. FIBULA
15. PATELLA
16. PHALANGES
17. METATARSUS
18. HUMERUS
19. RADIUS
20. ULNA
21. CARPUS
22. METACARPUS

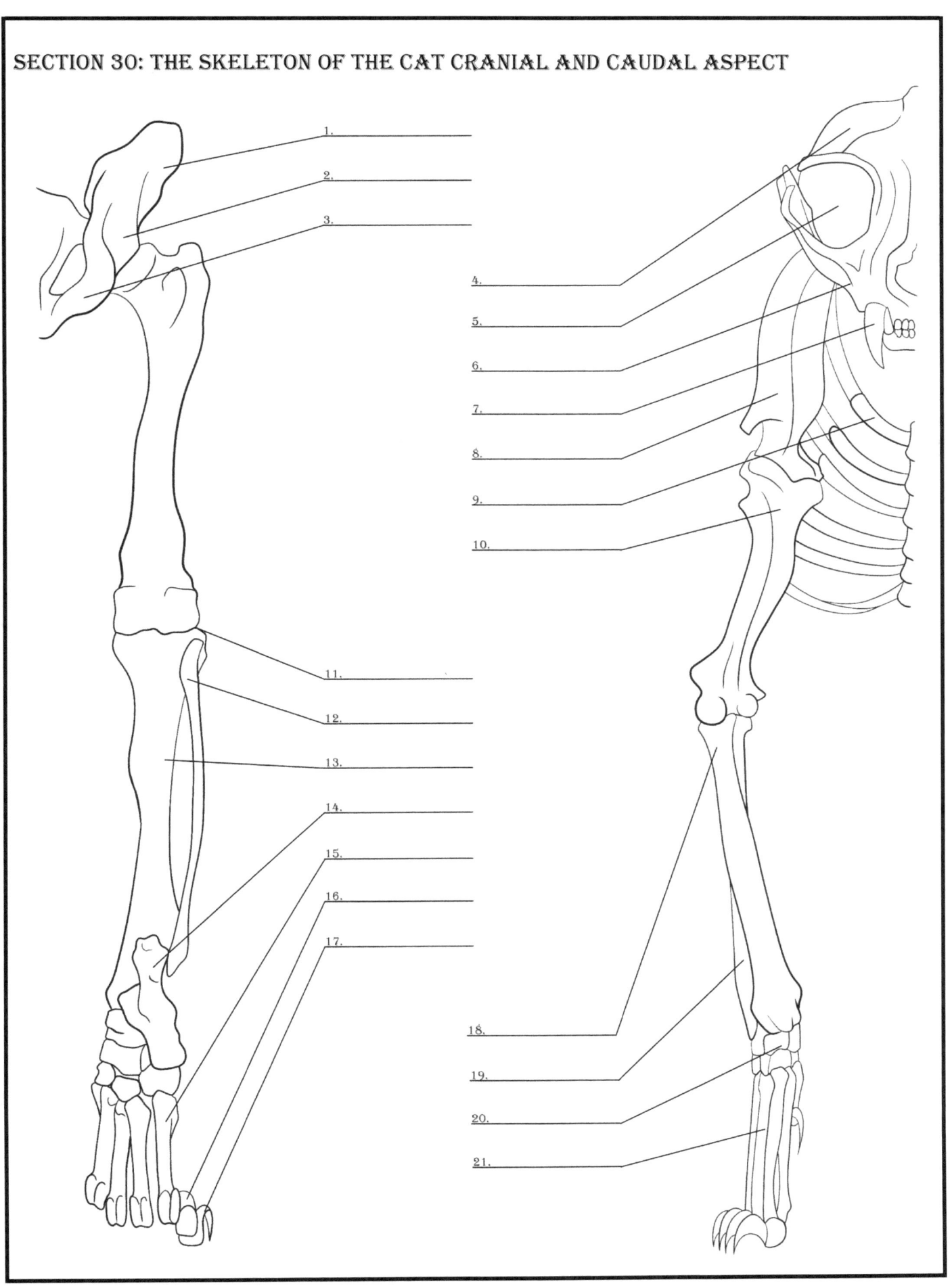

1.
2.
3.
4.
5.
6.
7.
8.
9.
10.
11.
12.
13.
14.
15.
16.
17.
18.
19.
20.
21.

SECTION 30: THE SKELETON OF THE CAT CRANIAL AND CAUDAL ASPECT

1. HIPBONE
2. HIP JOINT
3. ISCHIATIC TUBERCLE
4. SKULL
5. ORBIT
6. MANDIBLE
7. CANINE TOOTH
8. SCAPULA
9. RIB
10. HUMERUS
11. STIFLE JOINT
12. FIBULA
13. TIBIA
14. CALCANEAN BONE
15. METATARSAL BONE
16. PHALANGEAL BONE
17. CLAW BONE

SECTION 31: THE SKELETON OF THE CAT DORSAL ASPECT

1. _____

2. _____

3. _____

4. _____

5. _____

6. _____

7. _____

8. _____

9. _____

10. _____

SECTION 31: THE SKELETON OF THE CAT DORSAL ASPECT

1. ORBIT
2. SKULL
3. ATLAS
4. AXIS
5. SCAPULA
6. HUMERUS
7. RIB
8. SACRUM
9. ILIUM
10. ISCHIUM

SECTION 32: THE MUSCLES OF THE CAT LATERAL ASPECT

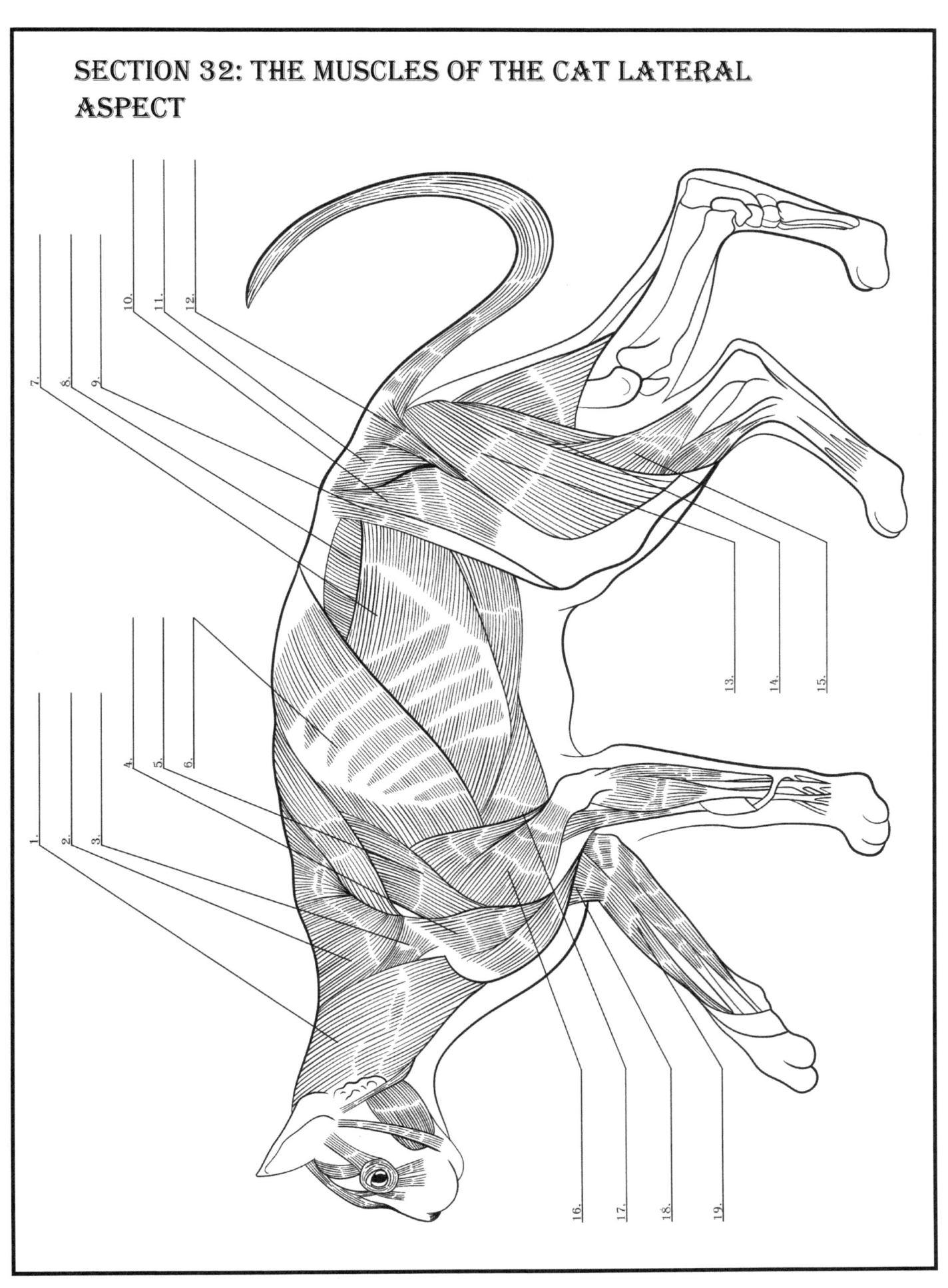

SECTION 32: THE MUSCLES OF THE CAT LATERAL ASPECT

1. BRAHIOCEPHALICUS MUSCLE
2. TRAPEZIUS MUSCLE
3. OMOSTRANSVERSARIUS MUSCLE
4. DELTOIDEUS MUSCLE
5. INFRASPINATUSM MUSCLE
6. LATISSIMUS DORSI MUSCLE
7. EXTERNAL OBLIQUE ABDOMINAL MUSCLE
8. INTERNAL OBLIQUE ABDOMINAL MUSCLE
9. SARTORIUS MUSCLE
10. TENSOR FASCIAE LATAE MUSCLE
11. CAUDOFEMORALIS MUSCLE
12. SERRATUS VENTRALIS MUSCLE
13. BICEPS FEMORIS MUSCLE
14. SEMITENDINOSUS MUSCLE
15. GASTROCNEMICUS MUSCLE
16. TRICEPS BRACHII MUSCLE
17. PECTORALIS PROFUNDUS MUSCLE
18. PECTORALIS DESCENDENS MUSCLE
19. EXTENSOR CARPI RADIALIS

SECTION 33: THE MUSCLES OF THE CAT CRANIAL AND CAUDAL ASPECT

1. _____

2. _____

3. _____

4. _____

5. _____

6. _____

7. _____

8. _____

9. _____

10. _____

11. _____

12. _____

13. _____

14. _____

15. _____

16. _____

17. _____

18. _____

19. _____

20. _____

21. _____

22. _____

23. _____

24. _____

25. _____

SECTION 33: THE MUSCLES OF THE CAT CRANIAL AND CAUDAL ASPECT

1. GLUTEUS SUPERFICIAL MUSCLE
2. CAUDOFEMORALIS MUSCLE
3. BICEPS FEMORIS MUSCLE
4. SEMITENDINOSUS MUSCLE
5. SEMIMEMBRANOSUS MUSCLE
6. GRACILIS MUSCLE
7. TRAPEZIUS MUSCLE
8. BRACHIOCEPHALICUS MUSCLE
9. STERNOHYOIDEUS MUSCLE
10. OMOTRANSVERSARIUS MUSCLE
11. DELTOIDEUS MUSCLE
12. CLEIDOBRACHIALIS MUSCLE
13. PECTORALES MUSCLE
14. GASTROCNEMICUS MUSCLE
15. FLEXORES DIGITORUM PROFUNDI MUSCLE
16. EXTENSOR DIGITORUM MUSCLE
17. FLEXOR DIGITORUM SUPERFICIALIS MUSCLE
18. INTEROSSEI PLANTARES MUSCLE
19. TRICEPS BRACHII MUSCLE
20. EXTENSOR DIGITORUM COMMUNIS MUSCLE
21. PRONATOR TERES MUSCLE
22. EXTENSOR CARPI RADIALIS & BRACHIORADIALIS MUSCLE
23. EXTENSOR DIGITORUM LATERALIS MUSCLE
24. FLEXOR CARPI RADIALIS MUSCLE
25. ABDUCTOR DIGITI IST MUSCLE

SECTION 34: THE MUSCLES OF THE CAT VENTRAL ASPECT

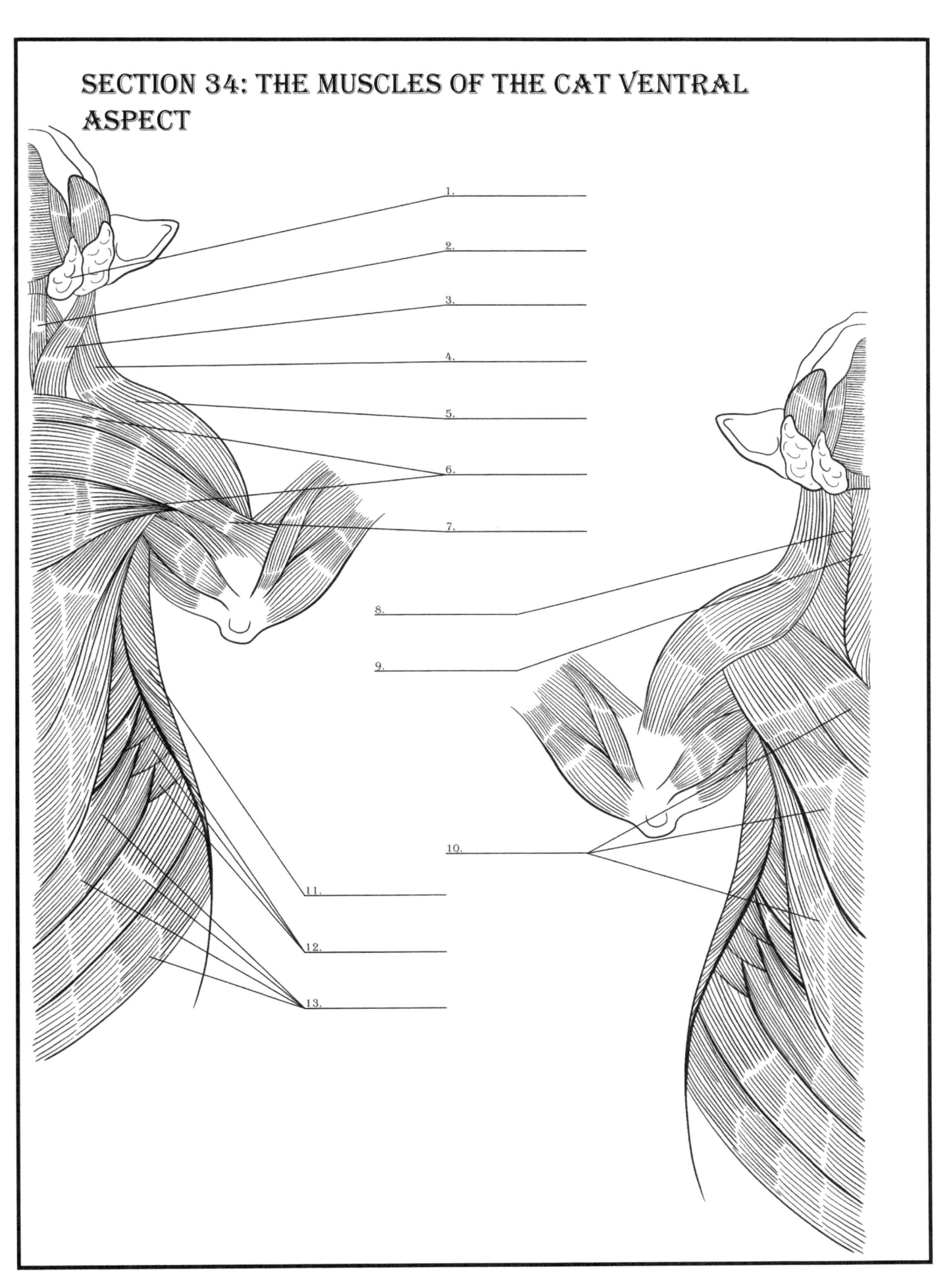

1. _____

2. _____

3. _____

4. _____

5. _____

6. _____

7. _____

8. _____

9. _____

10. _____

11. _____

12. _____

13. _____

SECTION 34: THE MUSCLES OF THE CAT VENTRAL ASPECT

1. MANDIBULAR GLAND
2. STERNOHPYOIDEUS MUSCLE
3. STERNOCEPHALICUS MUSCLE
4. CLEIDOCEPHALICUS, PARS CERVICALIS MUSCLE
5. CLEIDOCEPHALICUS, PARS MASTOIDEA MUSCLE
6. PECTORALIS TRANSVERSUS MUSCLE
7. PECTORALIS DESCENDENS MUSCLE
8. LONGUS CAPITIS MUSCLE
9. LONGUS COLLI MUSCLE
10. PECTORALIS PROFUNDUS MUSCLE
11. LATISSIMUS DORSI MUSCLE
12. SERRATUS VENTRALIS MUSCLE
13. OBLIQUUS EXTERNES ABDOMENS MUSCLE

SECTION 35: THE MUSCLES OF THE CAT DORSAL ASPECT

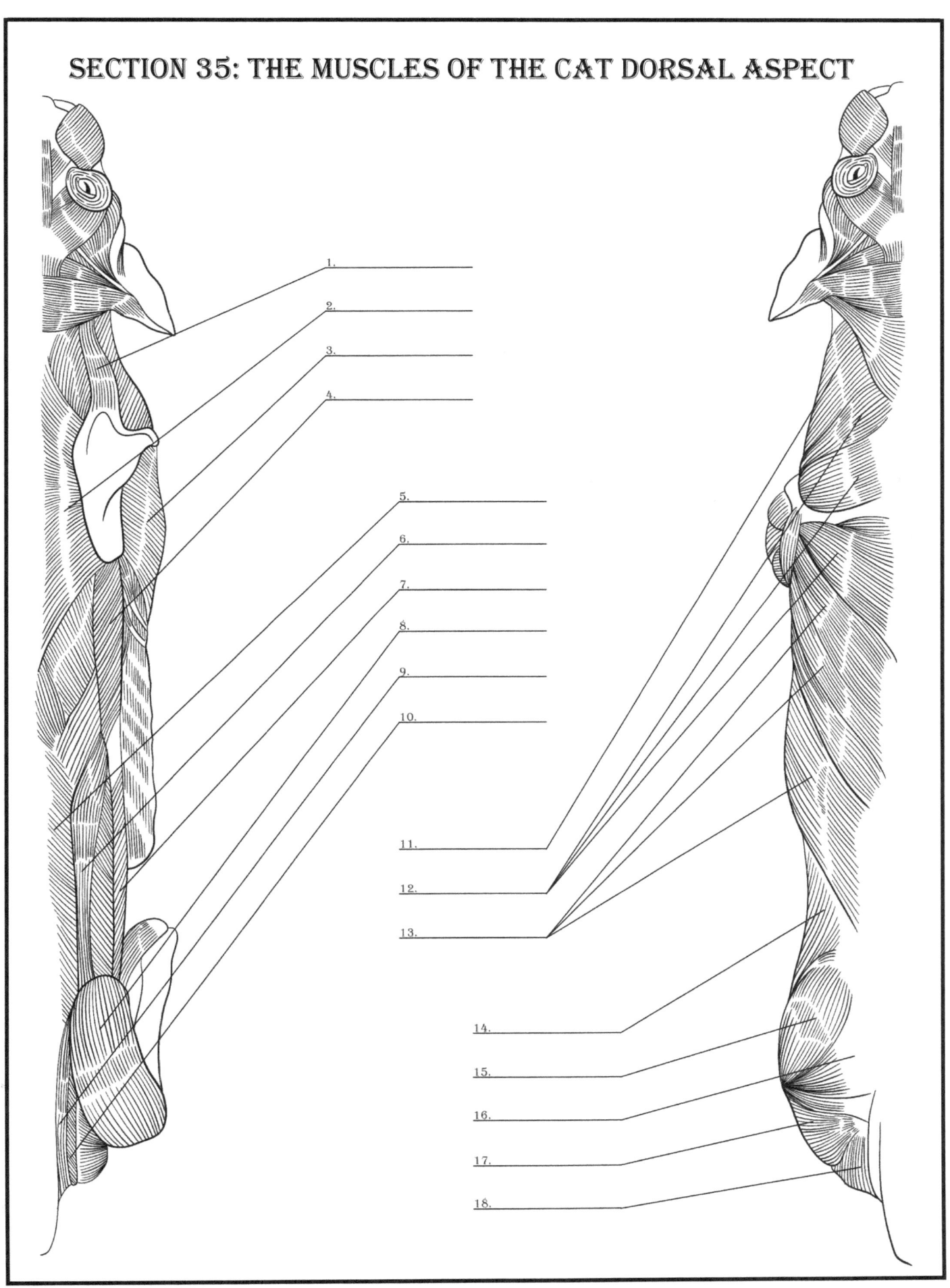

1.

2.

3.

4.

5.

6.

7.

8.

9.

10.

11.

12.

13.

14.

15.

16.

17.

18.

SECTION 35: THE MUSCLES OF THE CAT DORSAL ASPECT

1. RHOMBOIDEUS CAPITAIS MUSCLE
2. RHOMBOIDEUS THORACIS MUSCLE
3. SERRATUS VENTRALIS MUSCLE
4. LONGISSIMUS THORACIS MUSCLE
5. TRANSVERSOSPINALIS MUSCLE
6. LONGISSIMUS LUMBORUM MUSCLE
7. ILIOCOSTALIS LUMBORUM MUSCLE
8. GLUTEUS MEDIUS MUSCLE
9. SACROCAUDALIS DORSALIS MEDIALIS MUSCLE
10. SACROCAUDALIS DORSALIS LATERALIS MUSCLE
11. BRACHIOCEPUHALICUS MUSCLE
12. TRAPEZIUS MUSCLE
13. LATISSIMUS DORSI MUSCLE
14. OBLIQUUS EXTERNUS ABDOMINIS MUSCLE
15. GLUTEUS MEDIUS MUSCLE
16. GLUTEUS SUPERFICIALIS MUSCLE
17. BICEPS FEMORIS MUSCLE
18. SEMITENDINOSUS MUSCLE

1.

2.

3.

4.

5.

6.

7.

8.

9.

10.

11.

12.

SECTION 36: INTERNAL ORGANS OF THE CAT

1. BRAIN
2. ESOPHAGUS
3. TRACHEA
4. SPINAL CORD
5. LUNGS
6. LIVER
7. STOMACH
8. SPLEEN
9. KIDNEY
10. COLON
11. BLADDER
12. HEART

SECTION 37: BLOOD VESSELS OF THE CAT

1.

2.

3.

4.

5.

6.

7.

8.

9.

10.

11.

12.

SECTION 37: BLOOD VESSELS OF THE CAT

1. CRANIAL VENA CAVA
2. HEART
3. AORTA
4. CAUDAL VENA CAVA
5. FEMORAL ARTERY
6. SAPHENOUS VEIN
7. SPLEEN
8. PORTAL VEINS
9. JUGULAR VEIN
10. CAROTID ARTERY
11. CEPHALIC VEIN
12. BRACHIAL ARTERY

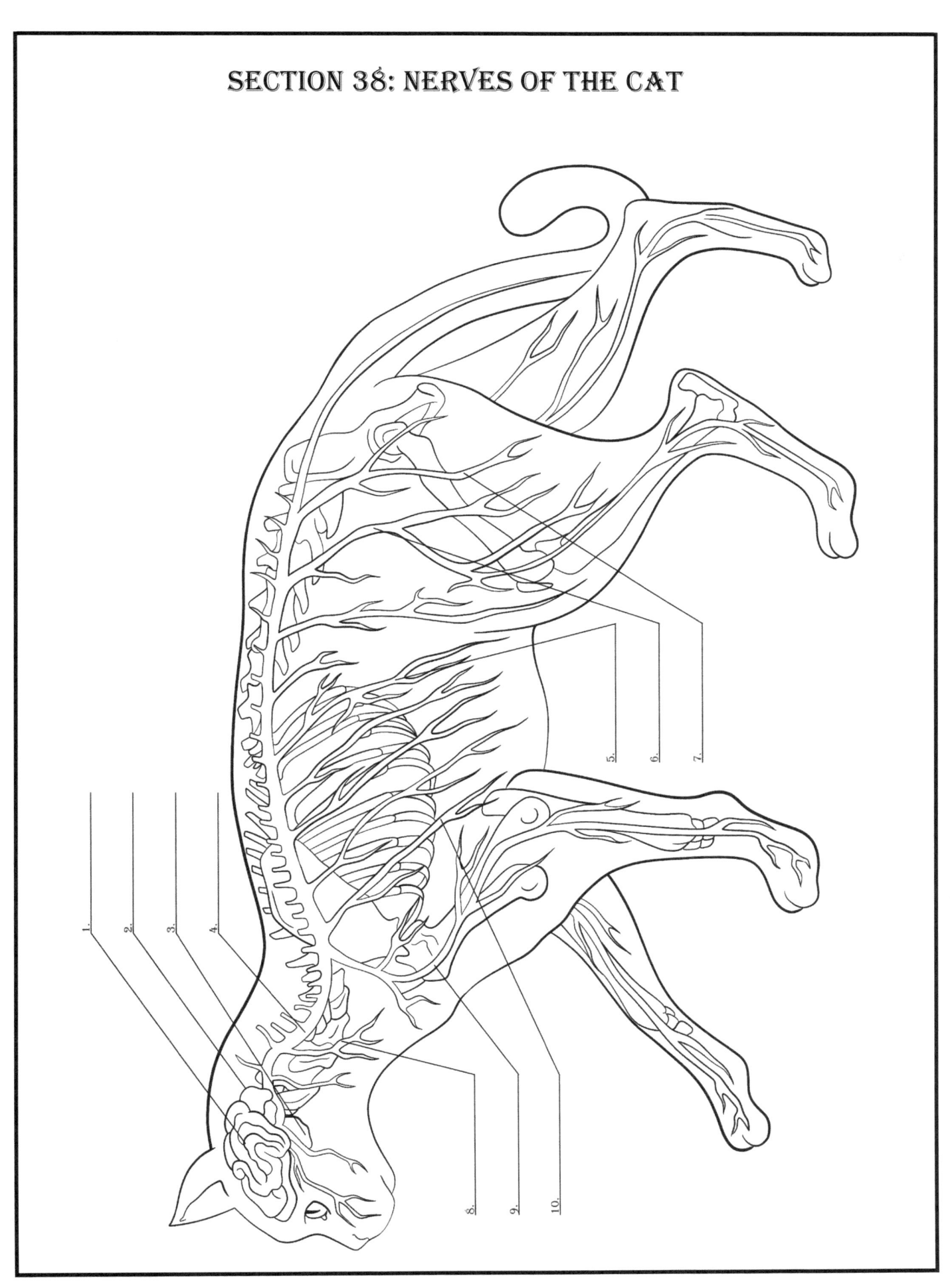

SECTION 38: NERVES OF THE CAT

1. CEREBRUM
2. CEREBELLUM
3. MEDULLA OBLONGATA
4. SPINAL CORD
5. THORACIC SPINAL
6. SCIATIC NERVE
7. FEMORAL NERVE
8. CERVICAL NERVE
9. RADIAL NERVE
10. THORACIC NERVE

SECTION 39: LUNGS OF THE CAT

1. _____

2. _____

3. _____

4. _____

5. _____

6. _____

7. _____

8. _____

9. _____

SECTION 39: RESPIRATORY SYSTEM OF THE CAT

1. RIGHT CRANIAL LOBE
2. LEFT CRANIAL LOBE
3. TRACHEA
4. LOBAR BRONCHUS
5. PRINCIPAL BRONCHUS
6. RIGHT MIDDLE LOBE
7. LEFT CAUDAL LOBE
8. RIGHT CAUDAL LOBE
9. ACCESSORY LOBE

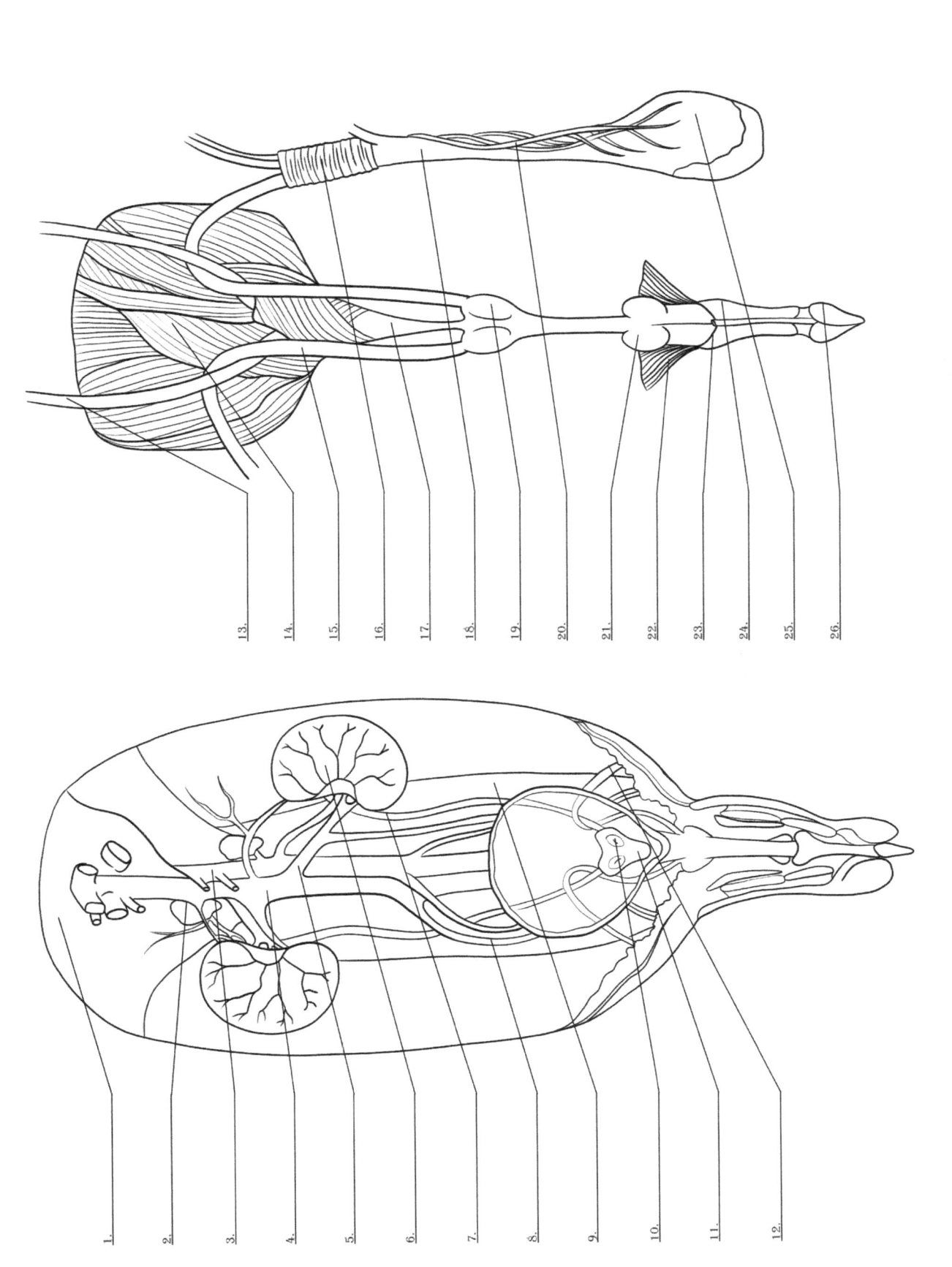

SECTION 40: UROGENITAL SYSTEM OF THE CAT 1

1. DIAPHRAGM
2. ADRENAL GLAND
3. ABDOMINAL AORTA
4. CAUDAL VENA CAVA
5. RENAL AORTA AND VEIN
6. KIDNEY
7. URETER
8. TESTICULAR AORTA AND VEIN
9. PSOAS MAJOR MUSCLE
10. ORIFICE OF URETER
11. VESICULAR TRIGONE
12. DUCTUS DEFERENS
13. URETER
14. URINARY BLADDER
15. DUCTUS DEFERENS
16. INGUINAL CANAL
17. NECK OF BLADDER
18. SPERMATIC CORD
19. PROSTATE GLAND
20. CREMASTER MUSCLE
21. BULBOURETHAL GLAND
22. ISCHIOCARVERNOSUS MUSCLE
23. BULBOSPONGIOSUS MUSCLE
24. BODY OF PENIS
25. TESTIS
26. GLANS PENIS

SECTION 41: UROGENITAL SYSTEM OF THE CAT 2

1. _____

2. _____

3. _____

4. _____

5. _____

6. _____

7. _____

8. _____

9. _____

10. _____

11. _____

12. _____

13. _____

14. _____

15. _____

16. _____

17. _____

18. _____

19. _____

20. _____

21. _____

22. _____

23. _____

24. _____

25. _____

26. _____

27. _____

28. _____

SECTION 41: UROGENITAL SYSTEM OF THE CAT 2

1. PAPILLA
2. KOSTIUM PAPILLARE
3. PAPILLARY DUCT
4. AMINIONIC MEMBRANE
5. FETUS
6. ZONARY PLACENTA
7. ALLANTONIC MEMBRANE
8. UMBILICAL CORD
9. CHORIONIC MEMBRANE
10. LATERAL THORACIC VEIN AND ARTERY
11. CAUDAL THORACIC MAMMA
12. CRANIAL ABDOMINAL MAMMA
13. CRANIAL SUPERFICIAL EPIGASTRIC VEIN AND ARTERY
14. CAUDAL ABDOMINAL MAMMA
15. INGUINAL MAMMA
16. CAUDAL SUPERFICIAL EPIGASTRIC VEIN AND AORTA
17. KIDNEY
18. URETER
19. SUSPENSORY LIGAMENT
20. OVARY
21. UTERINE HORN
22. BROAD LIGAMENT
23. RECTUM
24. URINARY BLADDER
25. VAGINA
26. PELVIC SYMPHIS
27. VESTIBULE
28. VULVA

SECTION 42: DIGESTIVE SYSTEM OF THE CAT 1

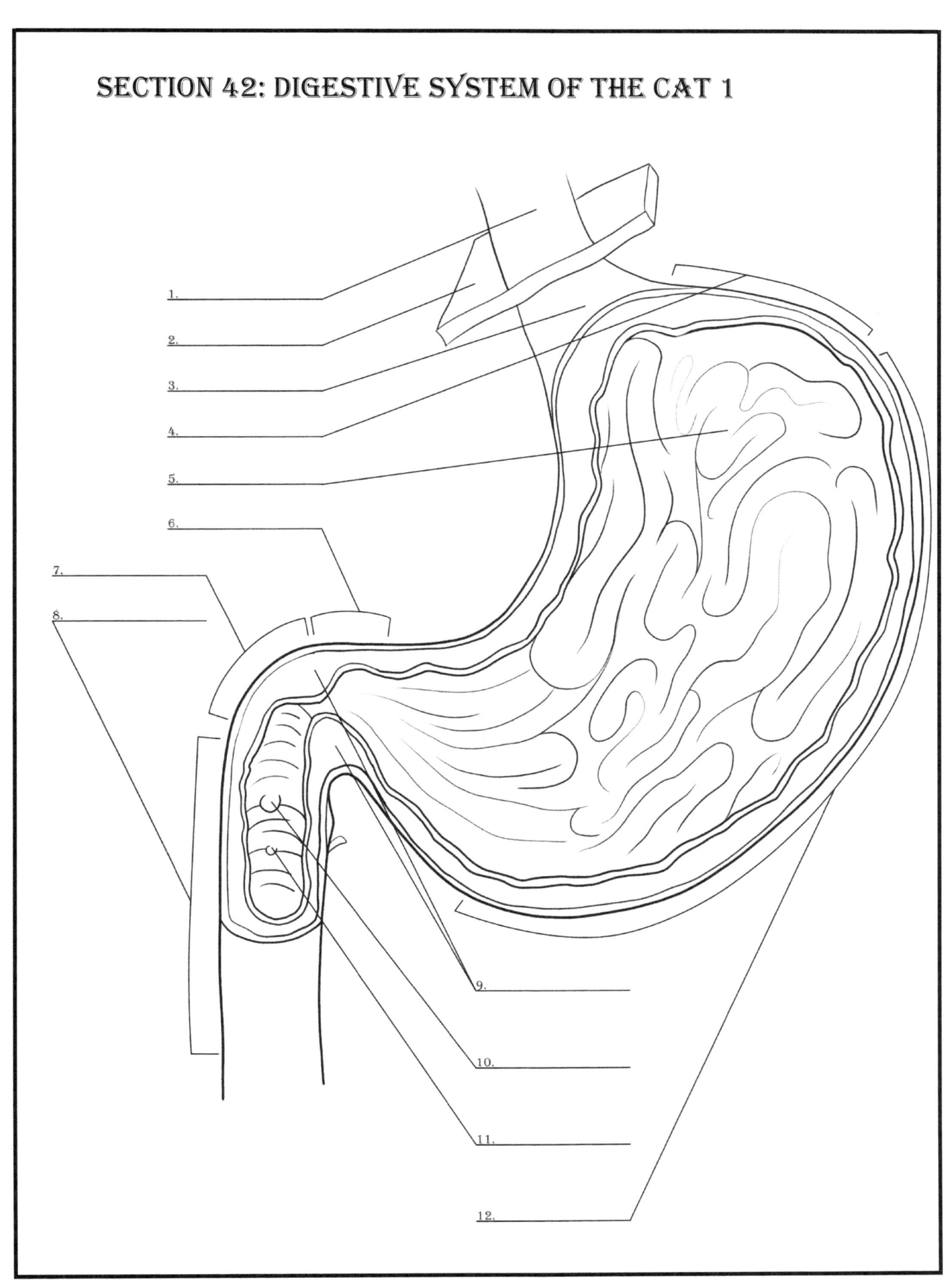

1. _____
2. _____
3. _____
4. _____
5. _____
6. _____
7. _____
8. _____
9. _____
10. _____
11. _____
12. _____

SECTION 42: DIGESTIVE SYSTEM OF THE CAT 1

1. ESOPHAGUS
2. DIAPHRAGM
3. CARDIA
4. FUNDUS
5. GASTRIC FOLDS
6. PYLORIC ANTRUM
7. PYLORIC CANAL
8. DESCENDING DUODENUM
9. PYLORIC SPINCTER
10. MAJOR DUODENAL PAPILLA
11. MINOR DUODENAL PAPILLA
12. BODY OF STOMACH

SECTION 43: DIGESTIVE SYSTEM OF THE CAT 2

1.

2.

3.

4.

5.

6.

7.

8.

9.

10.

11.

12.

13.

14.

15.

16.

17.

18.

19.

20.

21.

22.

SECTION 43: DIGESTIVE SYSTEM OF THE CAT 2

1. CAUDAL VENA CAVA
2. PORTAL VEIN
3. HEPATIC ARTERY
4. GALL BLADDER
5. LEFT LATERAL LOBE
6. PAPILLARY PROCESS OF CAUDATE LOBE
7. CAUDATE PROCESS OF CAUDATE LOBE
8. RIGHT LATERAL LOBE
9. RIGHT MEDIAL LOBE
10. QUADRATE LOBE
11. CAUDAL VENA CAVA
12. HEPATIC VEIN
13. CORONARY LIGAMENT
14. LEFT TRIANGULAR LIGAMENT
15. RIGHT TRIANGULAR LIGAMENT
16. RIGHT LATERAL LOBE
17. CAUDATE PROCESS
18. RIGHT MEDIAL LOBE
19. ROUND LIGAMENT OF LIVER
20. GALL BLADDER
21. LEFT MEDIAL LOBE
22. LEFT LATERAL LOBE

SECTION 44: THE SKULL OF THE CAT LATERAL ASPECT

SECTION 44: THE SKULL OF THE CAT LATERAL ASPECT

1. PREMAXILLA
2. NASAL BONE
3. MAXILLA
4. LACRIMAL BONE
5. ETHMOID
6. PALATINE BONE
7. ORBIT
8. FRONTAL BONE
9. PARIETAL BONE
10. TEMPORAL BONE
11. SAGITTAL CREST
12. EXTERNAL ACOUSTIC MEATUS
13. TYMPANIC BULLA
14. NUCHAL BREAST
15. OCCIPITAL BONE
16. OCCIPITAL CONDYLE
17. ZYGOMATIC BONE
18. TEMPOROMANDIBULAR JOINT
19. ANGULAR PROCESS OF MANDIBLE
20. MANDIBLE
21. UPPER FOURTH PREMOLAR
22. INFRAORBITAL FORAMEN
23. CARNASSIAL TOOTH
24. DENTARY
25. CANINE TOOTH
26. INCISOR TOOTH

SECTION 45: INSIDE THE SKULL OF THE CAT

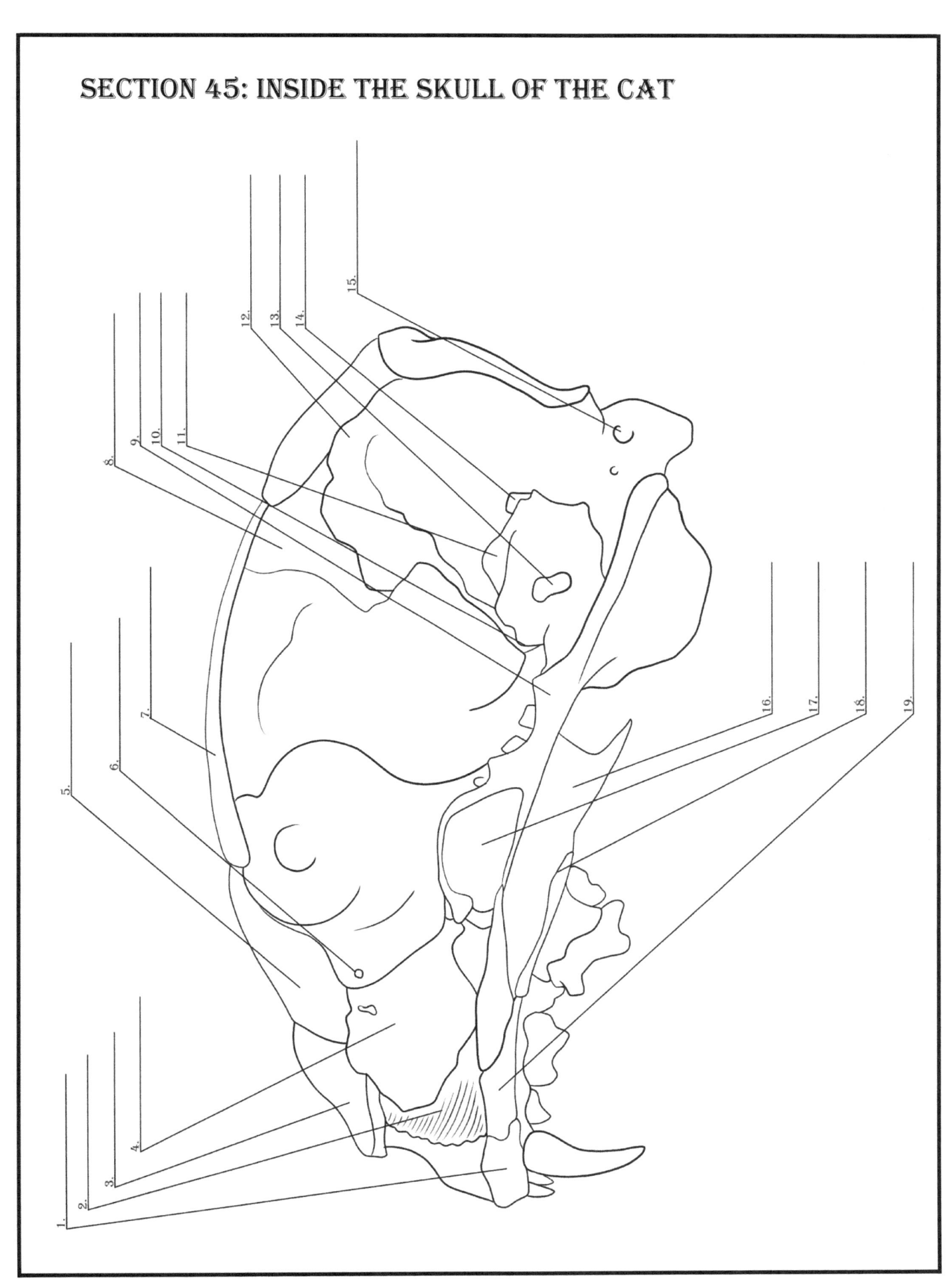

SECTION 45: INSIDE THE SKULL OF THE CAT

1. PREMAXILLA
2. TURBINALS
3. NASAL
4. ETHMOID
5. FRONTAL
6. CRIBIFORM PLATE
7. PARIETAL
8. TENTORIUM
9. TORSUM SELLAE
10. HIATUS FACIALIS
11. SUBARCUATE FOSSA
12. CEREBELLAR FOSSA
13. INTERNAL AUDITORY MEATUS
14. ENDOLYMPHATIC FORAMEN
15. CONDYLAR FORAMEN
16. HOMULUS
17. SPHENOIDAL SINUS
18. PALATINE
19. MAXILLA

SECTION 46: THE SKULL OF THE CAT DORSAL ASPECT

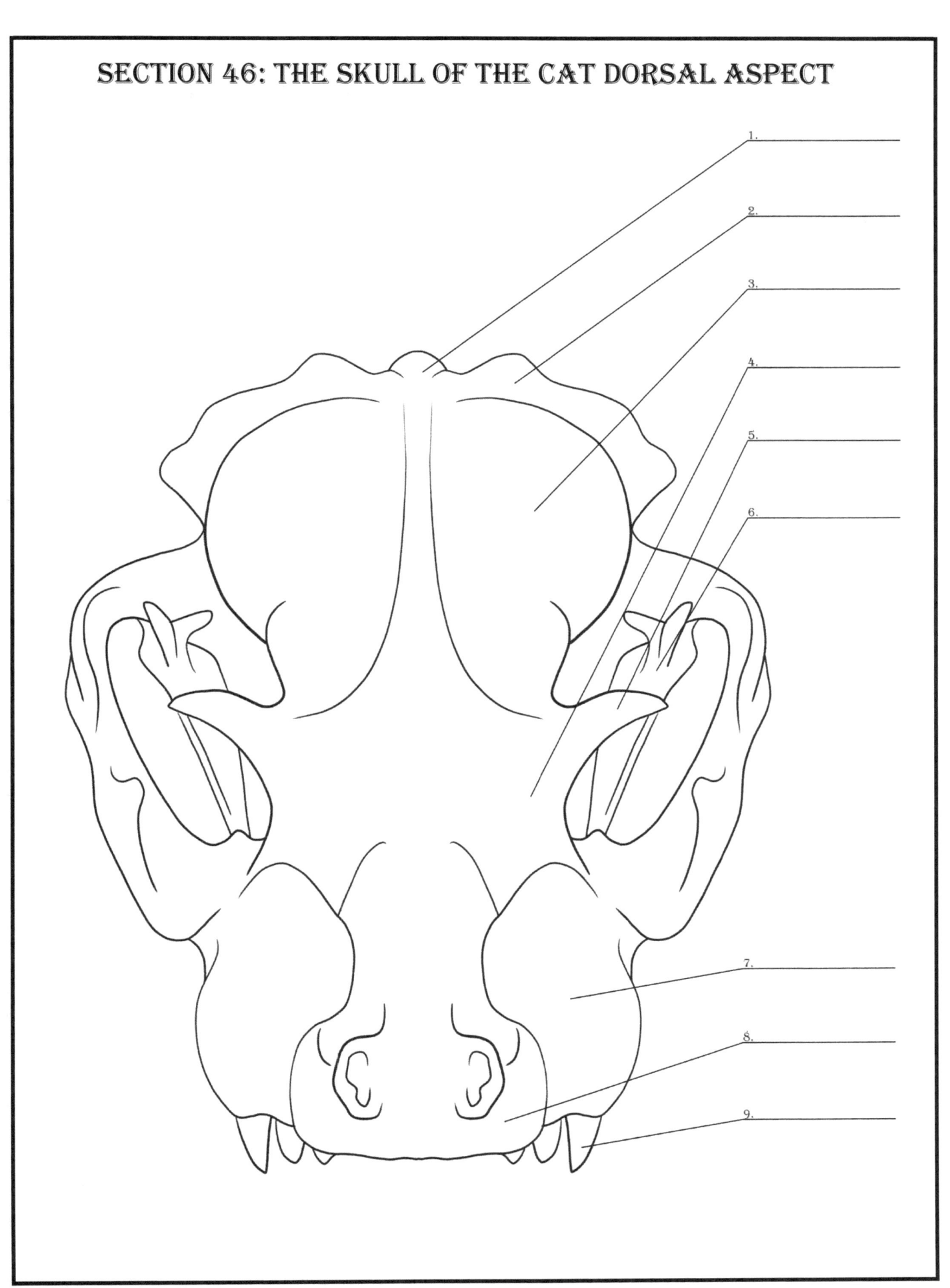

1. _____

2. _____

3. _____

4. _____

5. _____

6. _____

7. _____

8. _____

9. _____

SECTION 46: THE SKULL OF THE CAT DORSAL ASPECT

1. SAGITTAL CREST
2. LAMBDOIDAL RIDGE
3. PARIETAL
4. FRONTAL
5. POSTORBITAL PROCESS
6. MANDIBLE
7. MAXILLA
8. PREMAXILLA
9. CANINE TOOTH

SECTION 47: THE SKULL OF THE CAT VENTRAL ASPECT

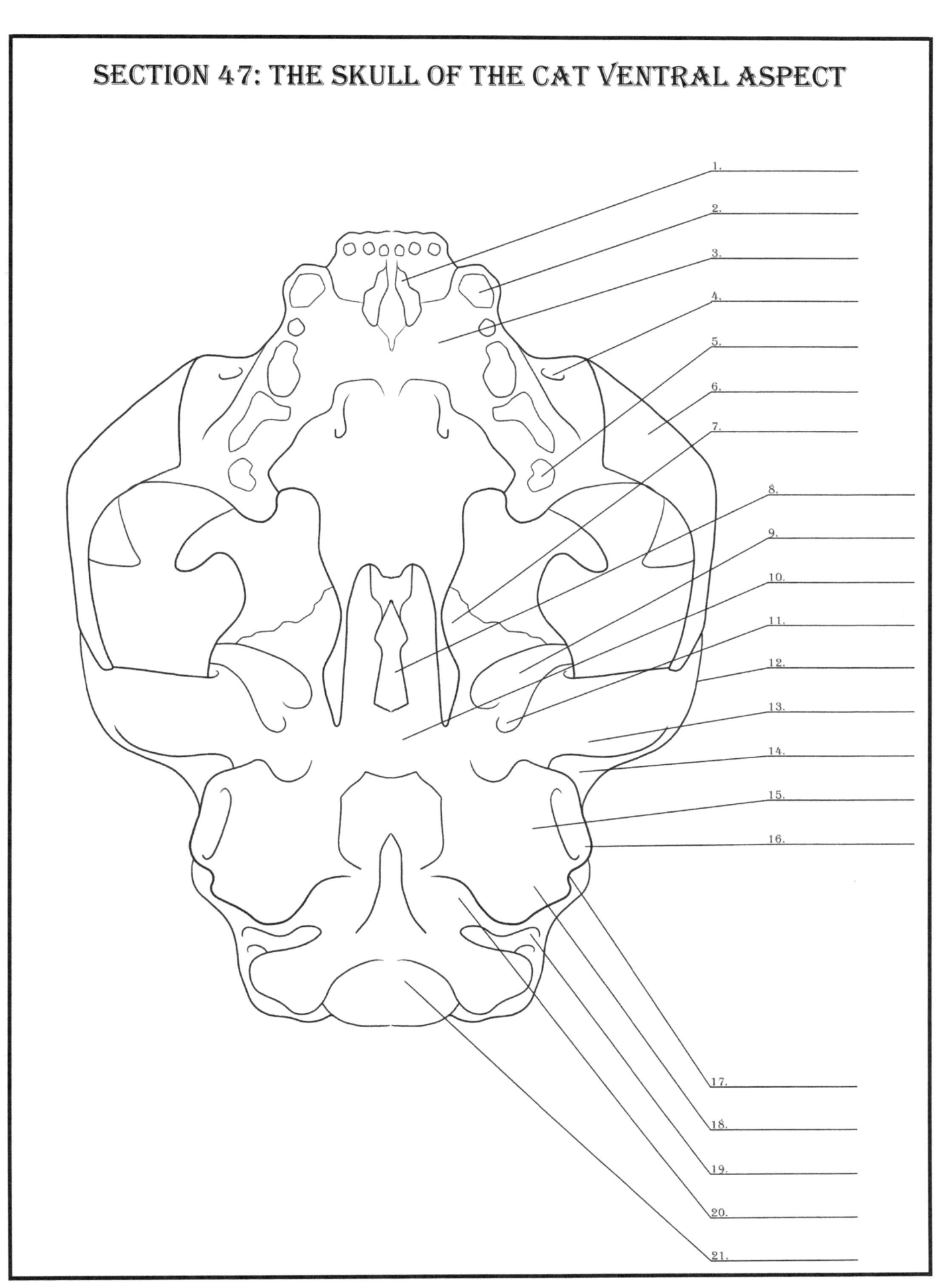

1.

2.

3.

4.

5.

6.

7.

8.

9.

10.

11.

12.

13.

14.

15.

16.

17.

18.

19.

20.

21.

SECTION 47: THE SKULL OF THE CAT VENTRAL ASPECT

1. INCISIVE FORAMEN
2. INCISOR TOOTH
3. PREMAXILLA
4. INFRAORBITAL FORAMEN
5. MOLAR TOOTH
6. MAXILLA
7. ORBITOSPHLENOID
8. PRESPHENOID
9. ALISPHLENOID
10. HYPOPHYSEAL FENESTRA
11. FORAMEN OVALE
12. ZYGOMATIC PROCESS
13. GLENOID FOSSA
14. POSTGLENOID PROCESS
15. TYMPANIC
16. STYLOMASTOID FORAMEN
17. MASTOID PROCESS
18. ENTOTYMPANIC
19. EXOCCIPITAL PROCESS
20. HYPOGLOSSAL FORAMEN
21. FORAMEN MAGNUM

SECTION 48: THE MUSCLES OF THE HEAD LATERAL ASPECT

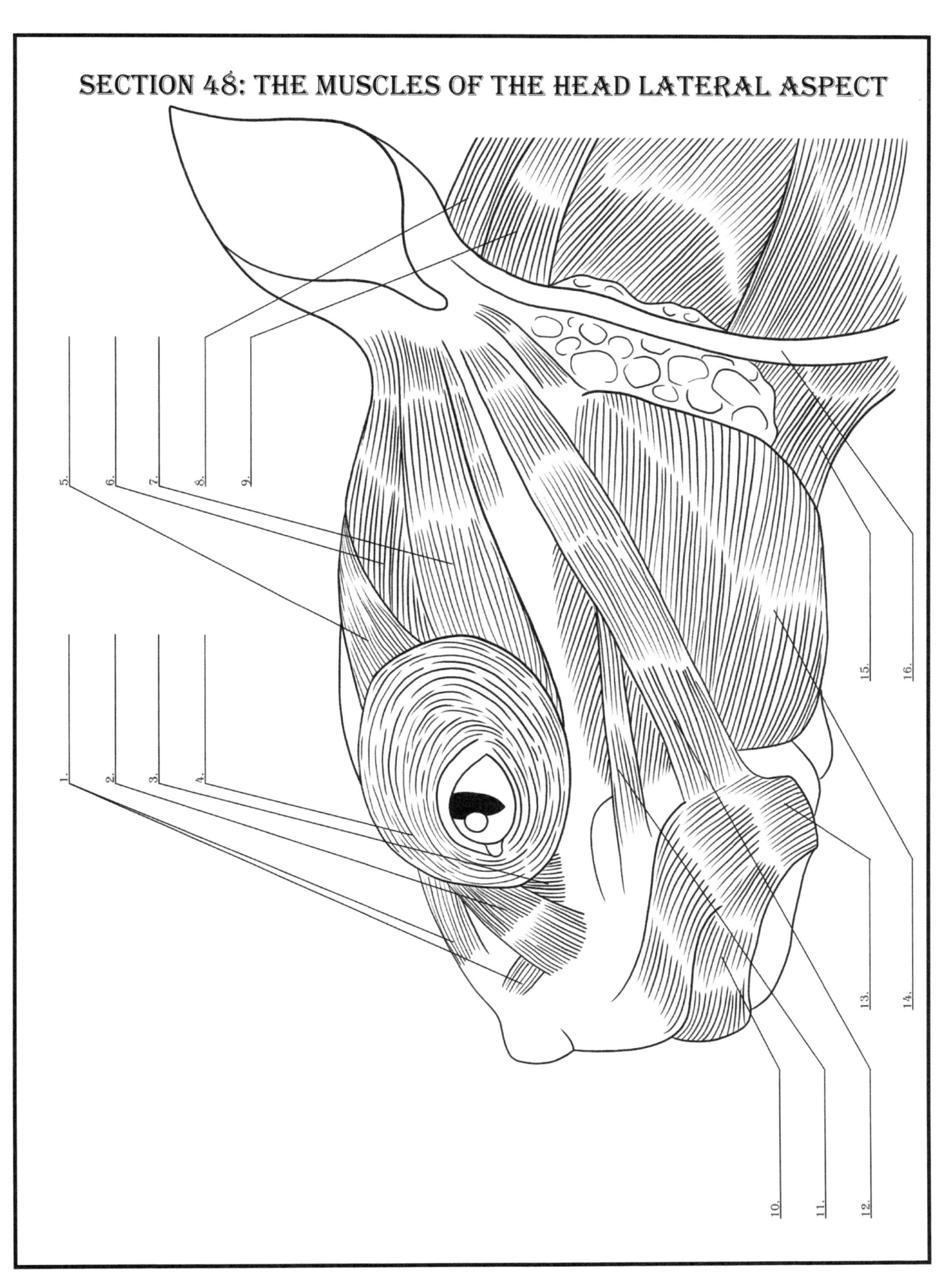

SECTION 48: THE MUSCLES OF THE HEAD LATERAL ASPECT

1. DORSALIS & LATERALIS NASI MUSCLES
2. LEVATOR NASOLABIALIS MUSCLE
3. MALARIS MUSCLE
4. ORBICULARIS OCULI MUSCLE
5. LEVATOR PALPEERDE SUPERIORIS MUSCLE
6. FRONTOSCUTULARIS MUSCLE
7. TEMPORALIS MUSCLE
8. CERVICOAURICULARIS PROFUNDUS MUSCLE
9. CERVICOAURICULARIS SUPERFICIALIS MUSCLE
10. ORBICULARIS ORIS MUSCLE
11. DEPRESSOR LABII MAXILLARIS MUSCLE
12. ZYGOMATICUS MUSCLE
13. DEPRESSOR LABII MANDIBULARIS MUSCLE
14. MASSETER MUSCLE
15. STERNOHPYOIDEUS MUSCLE
16. PARTOIDEOAURICULARIS MUSCLE

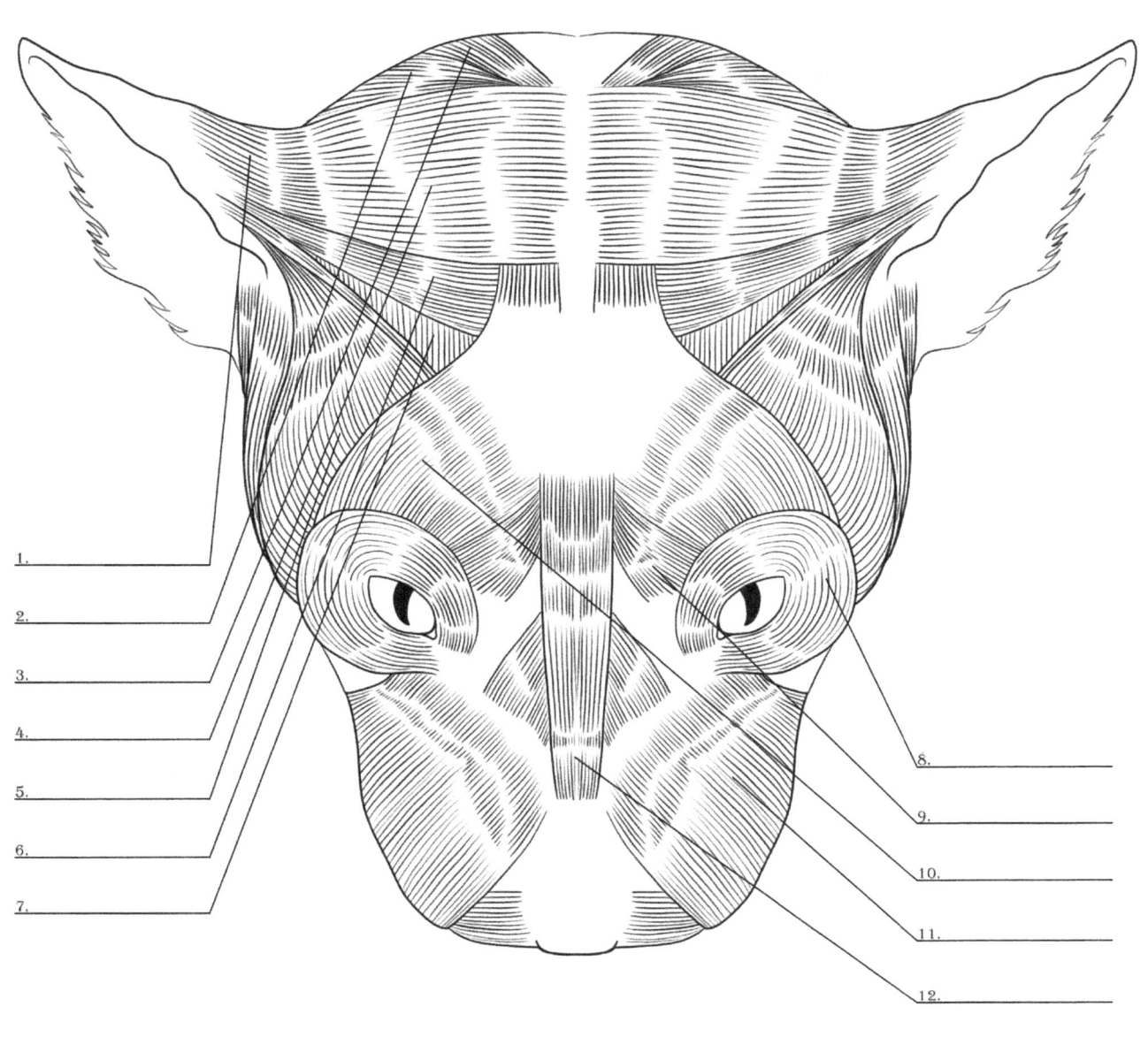

1.

2.

3.

4.

5.

6.

7.

8.

9.

10.

11.

12.

SECTION 49: THE MUSCLES OF THE HEAD DORSAL ASPECT

1. SCUTULOAURICULARIS PROFUNDUS MUSCLE
2. CERVICOAURICULARIS SUPERFICIALIS MUSCLE
3. CERVICOAURICULARIS PROFUNDUS MUSCLE
4. INTERSCUTULARIS MUSCLE
5. ZYGOMATICOAURICULARIS MUSCLE
6. PARIETOSCUTULARIS MUSCLE
7. TEMPORALIS MUSCLE
8. ORBICULARIS OCULI MUSCLE
9. LEVATOR OF THE MEDIAL EYE ANGLE
10. LEVATOR PALPEBRAE SUPERIORIS MUSCLE
11. LEVATOR NASOLABIALIS MUSCLE
12. DORSALIS NASI MUSCLE

SECTION 50: THE BRAIN OF THE CAT

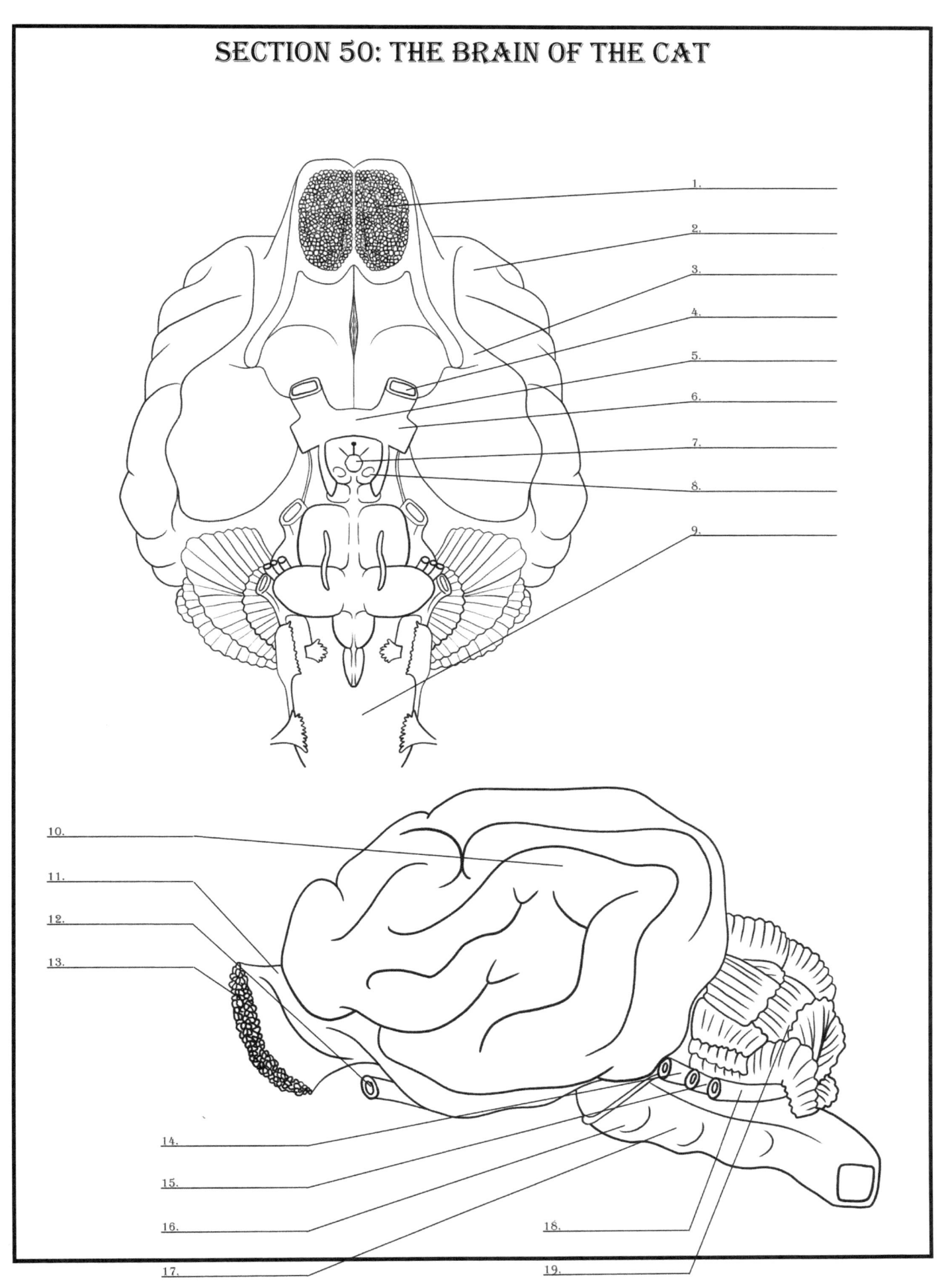

1. _____

2. _____

3. _____

4. _____

5. _____

6. _____

7. _____

8. _____

9. _____

10. _____

11. _____

12. _____

13. _____

14. _____

15. _____

16. _____

17. _____

18. _____

19. _____

SECTION 50: THE BRAIN OF THE CAT

1. OLFACTORY BULB
2. CEREBRAL HEMISPHERE
3. OLFACTORY TRACT
4. OPTIC NERVE
5. OPTIC CHIASM
6. OPTIC TRACT
7. HYPOPHYSIS
8. MAMMILLARY BODIES
9. MEDULLA
10. CEREBRAL HEMISPHERE
11. OLFACTORY TRACT
12. OPTIC NERVE
13. OLFACTORY BULB
14. TRIGEMINAL NERVE
15. FACIAL NERVE
16. PONS
17. VESTIBULOCOCHLEAR NERVE
18. CEREBELLAR HEMISPHERE

SECTION 51: THE EYE OF THE CAT

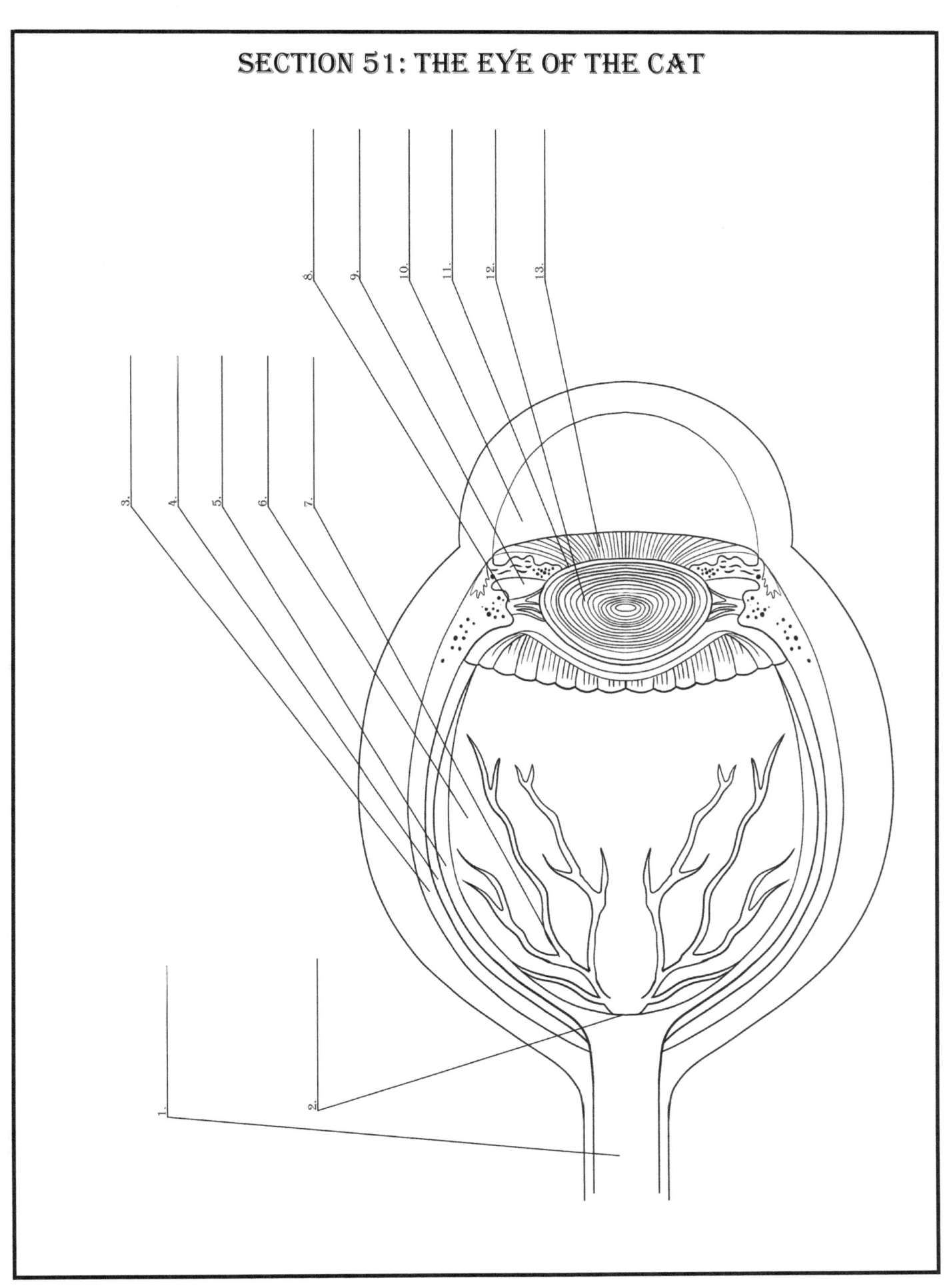

SECTION 51: THE EYE OF THE CAT

1. OPTIC NERVE
2. OPTIC DISC
3. CHOROID
4. TAPETUM LUCIDUM
5. RETINA
6. VITREOUS HUMOR
7. ARTERY
8. CILIARY BODY
9. POSTERIOR CHAMBER
10. ANTERIOR CHAMBER
11. PUPIL
12. LENS
13. IRIS

SECTION 52: THE EAR OF THE CAT

1. _____
2. _____
3. _____
4. _____
5. _____
6. _____
7. _____
8. _____
9. _____
10. _____
11. _____
12. _____
13. _____
14. _____
15. _____
16. _____
17. _____
18. _____
19. _____
20. _____
21. _____
22. _____
23. _____
24. _____
25. _____
26. _____

SECTION 52: THE EAR OF THE CAT

1. SCAPHA
2. CONCHA
3. EXTERNAL EAR CANAL VERTICAL PART
4. TEMPORALIS MUSCLE
5. SKULL
6. EXTERNAL EAR CANAL VERTICAL PART
7. OSSEOUS SEMICIRCULAR CANALS
8. INCUS
9. MALLEUS
10. EAR OSSICLE
11. PETROUS TEMPORAL BONE
12. OSSEOUS VESTIBULE
13. OSSEOUS COCHLEA
14. PETROUS TEMPORAL BONE
15. TYMPANIC MEMBRANE
16. AUDITORY TUBE
17. TYMPANIC BULLA
18. ANNULAR CARTILAGE
19. SHORT CRUS
20. INCUS
21. HEAD
22. LONG CRUS
23. MALLEUS
24. STAPES
25. BASE
26. MANUBRIUM

SECTION 53: THE HEART OF THE CAT

SECTION 53: THE HEART OF THE CAT

1. AORTIC ARCH
2. RIGHT ATRIUM
3. PULMONARY ARTERY
4. LEFT ATRIUM
5. RIGHT VENTRICLE
6. LEFT VENTRICLE
7. RIGHT VENTRICLE
8. PAPILLARY MUSCLE
9. CHORDA TENDINEA
10. VENTRICULAR SEPTUM
11. RIGHT VENTRICULAR FREE WALL
12. LEFT VENTRICLE
13. LEFT VENTRICULAR FREE WALL

SECTION 54: THORACIC LIMB

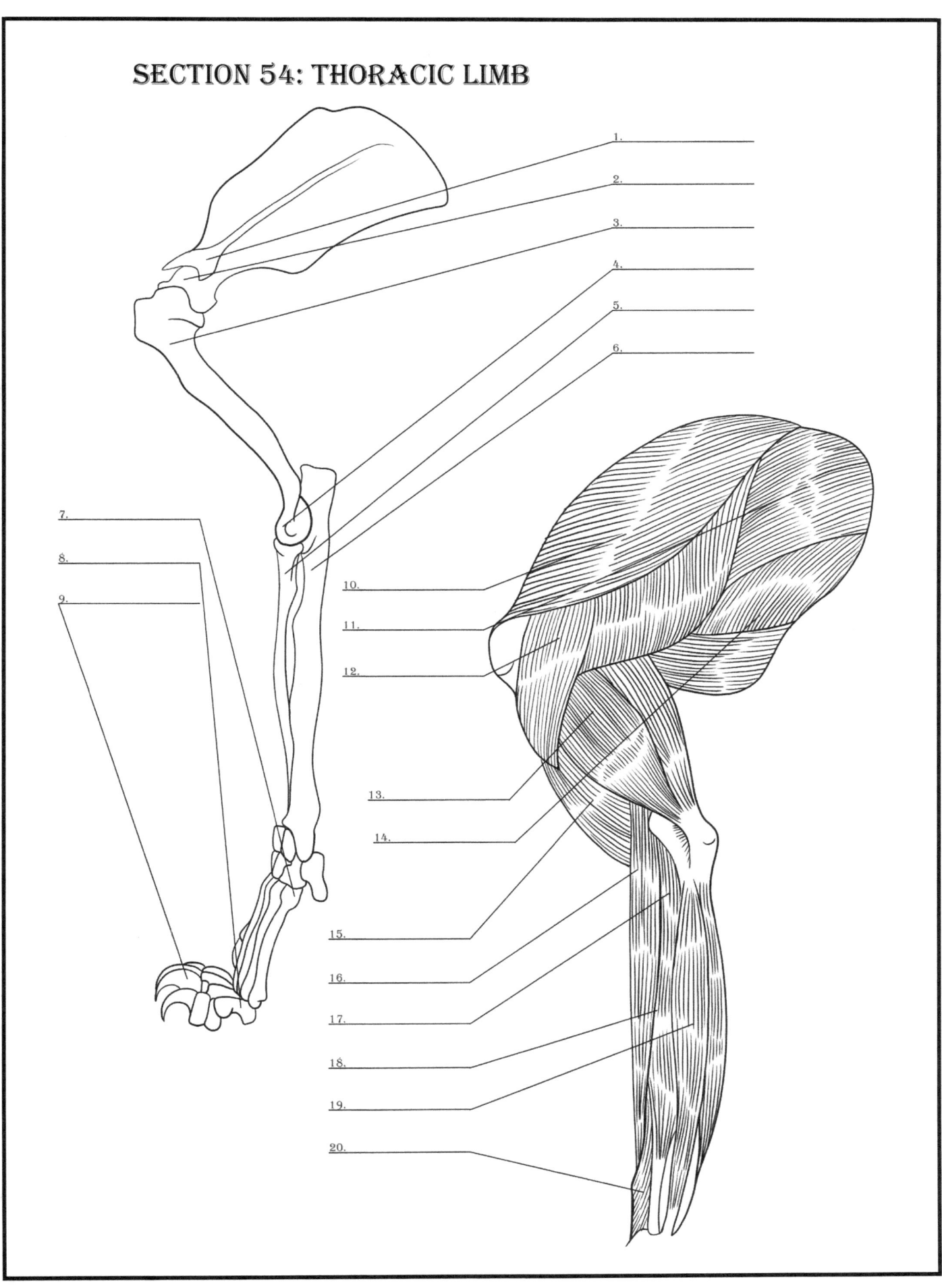

1.

2.

3.

4.

5.

6.

7.

8.

9.

10.

11.

12.

13.

14.

15.

16.

17.

18.

19.

20.

SECTION 54: THORACIC LIMB LATERAL ASPECT

1. PROCESS OF THE SHOULDER BLADE
2. SHOULDER JOINT
3. HUMERUS
4. ELBOW JOINT
5. RADIUS
6. ULNA
7. METACARPAL BONE
8. PHALANGEAL BONE
9. CLAW BONE
10. SUPRASPINATUS MUSCLE
11. INFRASPINATUSM MUSCLE
12. DELTOIDEUS MUSCLE
13. LATISSIMUS DORSI MUSCLE
14. TERES MAJOR MUSCLE
15. BICEPS BRACHII MUSCLE
16. BRACHIORADIALIS MUSCLE
17. EXTENSOR CARPI RADIALIS MUSCLE
18. EXTENSOR DIGITORUM COMMUNIS MUSCLE
19. EXTENSOR DIGITORUM LATERALIS MUSCLE
20. ABDUCTOR DIGITI IST MUSCLE

SECTION 55: PELVIC LIMB

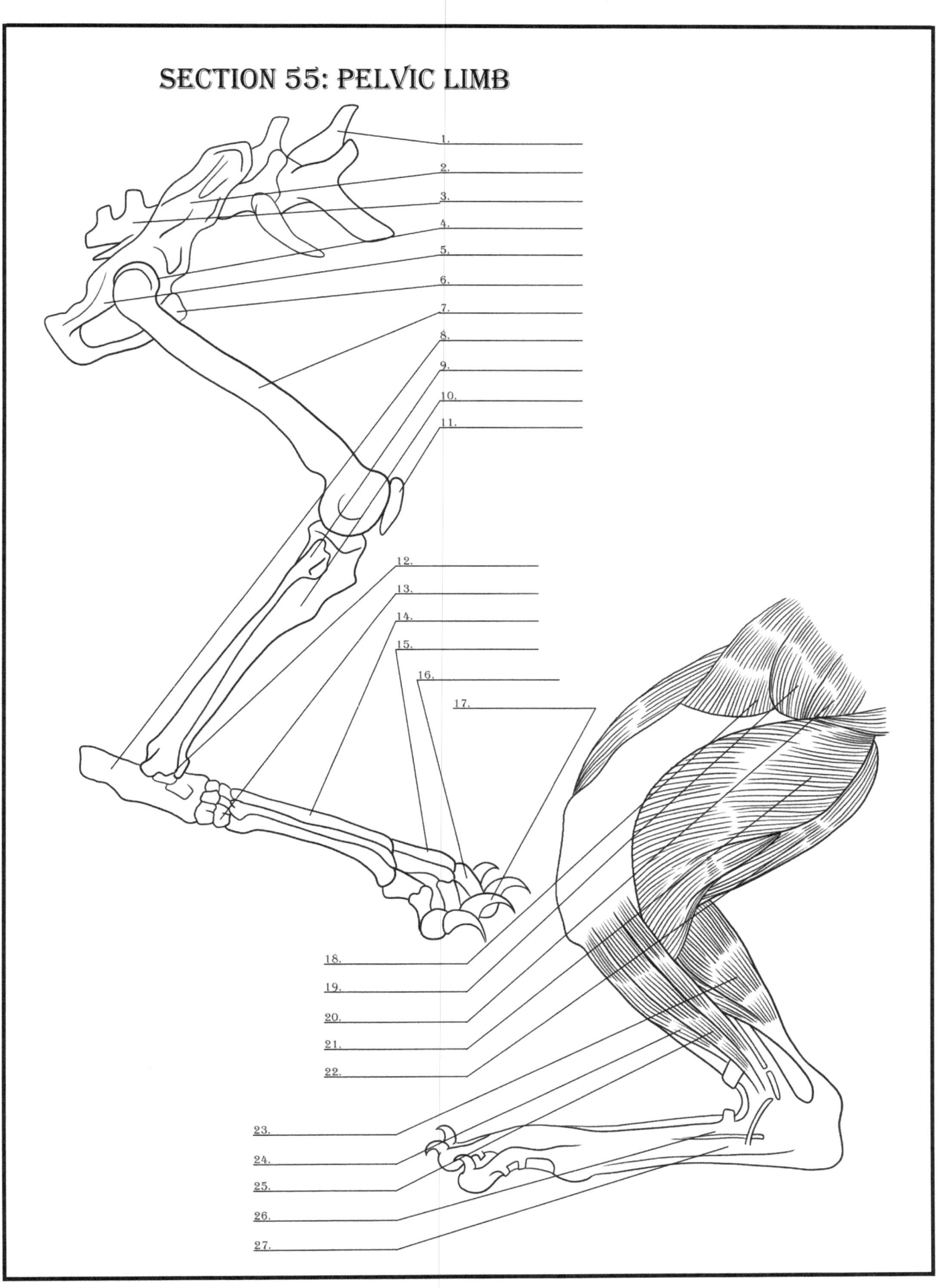

1.
2.
3.
4.
5.
6.
7.
8.
9.
10.
11.
12.
13.
14.
15.
16.
17.
18.
19.
20.
21.
22.
23.
24.
25.
26.
27.

SECTION 55: PELVIC LIMB

1. LAST LUMBAR VERTEBRA
2. HIP BONE
3. SACRUM
4. HIP JOINT
5. ISCHIAL BONE
6. PUBIC BONE
7. FEMUR
8. CALCANEUS
9. FIBULA
10. TIBIA
11. PATELLA
12. DISTAL TIBIO-FIBULAR JOINT
13. TARSAL BONE
14. METATARSAL BONE
15. PROXIMAL PHALANGEAL BONE
16. MIDDLE PHALANGEAL BONE
17. CLAW BONE
18. TENSOR FASCIAE LATAE MUSCLE
19. GLUTEUS MEDIUS MUSCLE
20. GLUTEUS SUPERFICIALIS MUSCLE
21. BICEPS FEMORIS MUSCLE
22. SEMITENDINOSUS MUSCLE
23. TRICEPS SURAE MUSCLE
24. TIBIALIS CRANIALIS MUSCLE
25. PERONEUS LONGUS MUSCLE
26. EXTENSOR DIGITORUM LONGUS MUSCLE
27. EXTENSOR DIGITORUM LATERALIS MUSCLE

SECTION 56: THE BONES OF THE FOOT 1

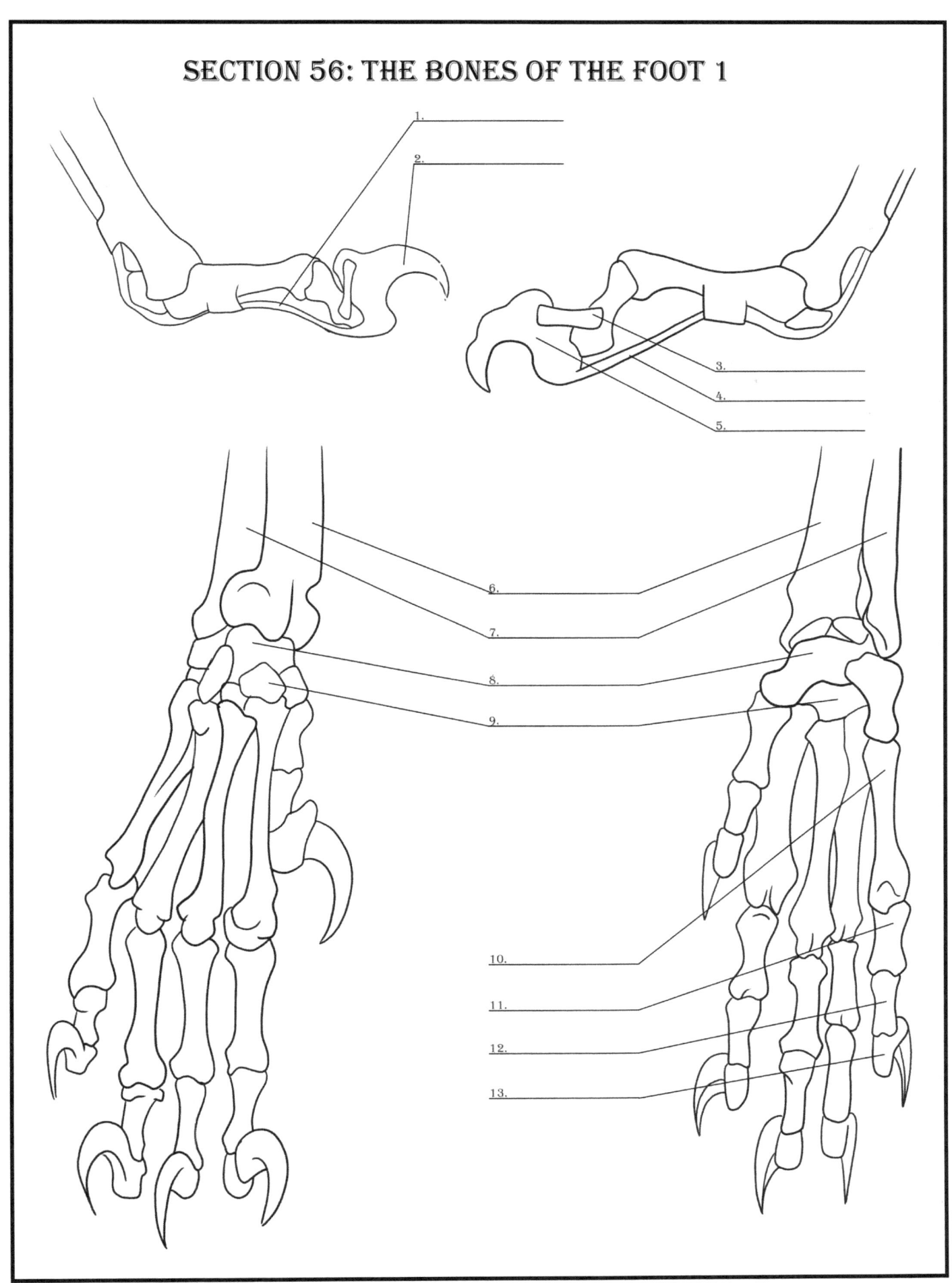

1. _____
2. _____
3. _____
4. _____
5. _____
6. _____
7. _____
8. _____
9. _____
10. _____
11. _____
12. _____
13. _____

SECTION 56: THE BONES OF THE FOOT 1

1. RELAXED TENDON
2. RETRACTED CLAW
3. LIGAMENT
4. TIGHTENED TENDON
5. EXTENDED CLAW
6. RADIUS
7. ULNA
8. PROXIMAL ROW OF CARPAL BONES
9. DISTAL ROW OF CARPAL BONES
10. METACARPAL BONE
11. PROXIMAL PHALANX
12. MIDDLE PHALANX
13. DISTAL PHALANX

SECTION 57: THE BONES OF THE FOOT 2

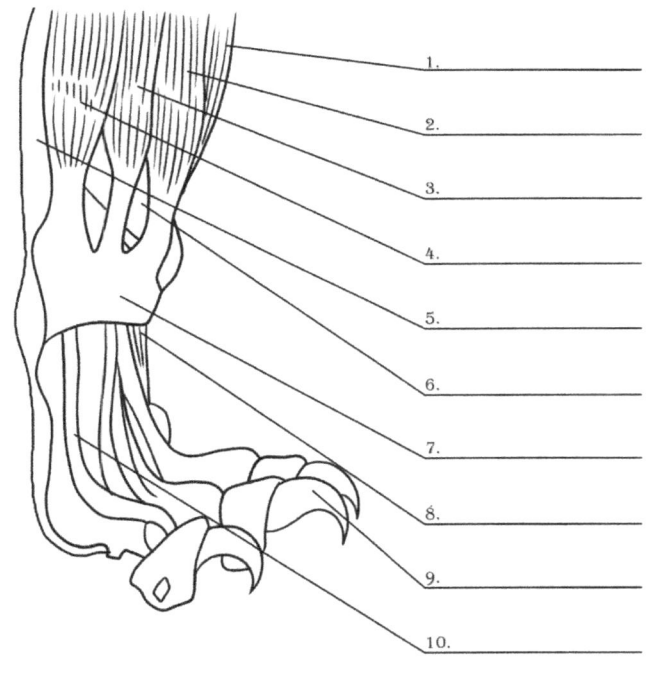

1. _____

2. _____

3. _____

4. _____

5. _____

6. _____

7. _____

8. _____

9. _____

10. _____

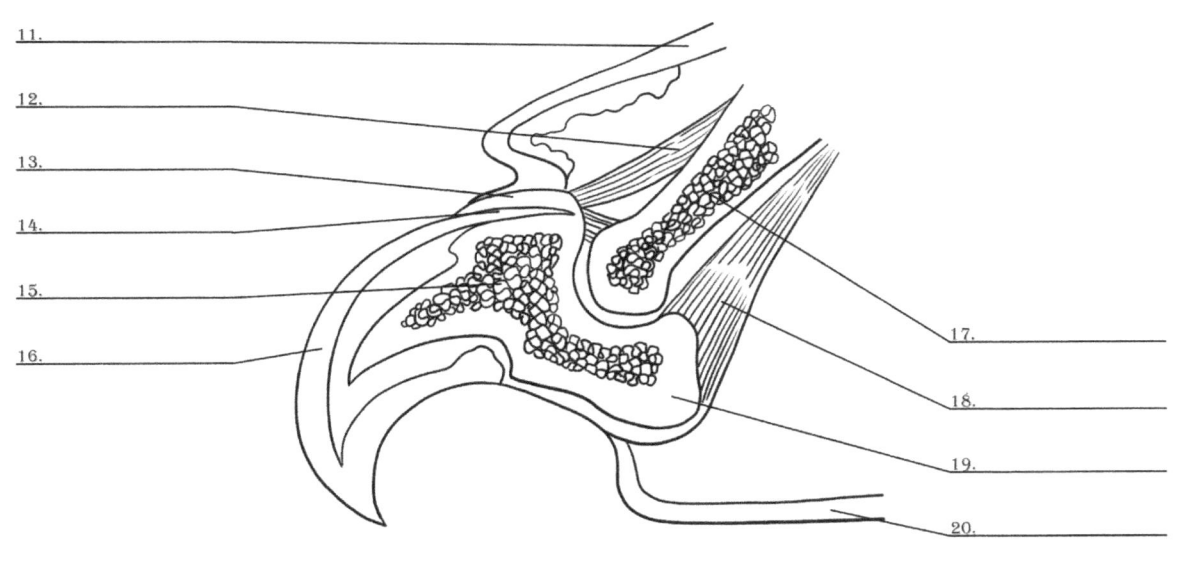

11. _____

12. _____

13. _____

14. _____

15. _____

16. _____

17. _____

18. _____

19. _____

20. _____

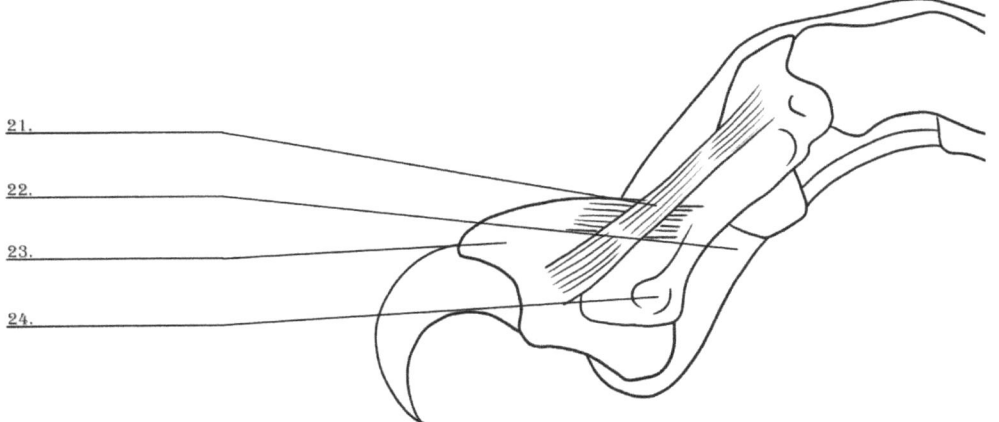

21. _____

22. _____

23. _____

24. _____

SECTION 57: THE BONES OF THE FOOT 2

1. EXTENSOR CARPI RADIALIS MUSCLE
2. COMMON DIGITAL EXTENSOR MUSCLE
3. LATERAL DIGITAL EXTENSOR MUSCLE
4. EXTENSOR CARPI ULNAS MUSCLE
5. FLEXOR CARPI ULNARIS
6. ABDUCTOR POLLICIS LINGUS MUSCLE
7. EXTENSOR RETINACULUM
8. TENDON OF MUSCLES EXTENSOR DIGITI
9. CLAW COVERING UNGICULAR PROCESS
10. DIGITAL EXTENSOR MUSCLE
11. SKIN OF CLAW SHEATH
12. COMBINED EXTENSOR TENDOUS
13. EXTENSOR PROCESS
14. UNGUICULAR CREST
15. UNGUICULAR PROCESS
16. CLAW
17. MIDDLE PHALANX
18. TENDON OF DEEP DIGITAL FLEXOR MUSCLE
19. FLEXOR TUBERCLE
20. DIGITAL PAD
21. TAUT ELASTIC LIGAMENT
22. TAUT DIGITAL FLEXOR TENDON
23. EXTENSOR PROCESS
24. PIVOT POINT